FOOD POWER

FOOD POWER

HOW FOODS CAN CHANGE YOUR MIND, YOUR PERSONALITY, AND YOUR LIFE

By
George
Schwartz, M.D.

McGRAW-HILL
BOOK COMPANY

New York
St. Louis
San Francisco
Düsseldorf
Mexico
Toronto

1 2 3 4 5 6 7 8 9 FGRFGR 7 8 3 2 1 0 9

LIBRARY OF CONGRESS CATALOGING IN PUBLICATION DATA

Schwartz, George R
Food power.
Bibliography: p.
Includes index.
1. Nutrition—Psychological aspects.   2. Human
behavior—Nutritional aspects.   3. Personality—
Nutritional aspects.   4. Food habits.   I. Title.
QP141.S348   613.2   78-32115
ISBN 0-07-055673-3

Book design by Roberta Rezk

This book is not intended to replace
the services of a physician. Any
application of the recommendations
set forth in the following pages
is at the reader's discretion and
sole risk.

To Patricia
whose spirit inspired and tamed me

ACKNOWLEDGMENTS

Over the past ten years, many people have been involved in the joyful labors of developing this book. I would like to thank some of the people who helped and without whom this book would not have been possible: my secretary and loyal friend, Pat Fredericks; my secretary, Anne Mc-Goey, who helped get the final manuscript in order; and Karen Sojka, whose help is appreciated. In the early stages, the guidance of Dr. A. Fritz was particularly important. Throughout, the wise counsel of Michael Masser helped me to continue with this work. The insights of Pamela, Peter, Rebekah, and Ruth were always valuable. And Ellen Levine told me to trust and it worked.

Contents

Preface

Several years ago I moved from a townhouse in a bustling city to a small red and white cottage deep in some woods nestled along a gently flowing river. I did not set out to imitate Thoreau, although closeness to nature's cycles brought me closer to my own rhythms.

I had not moved to find a hermitage. Instead, I was extremely busy with patients, administrative tasks, writing articles, helping edit a journal, and completing the major project of my professional life—editing a comprehensive textbook. I wanted to live apart from the distractions of city life in order to meet my worldly commitments and ever approaching deadlines.

After a few months I began to notice subtle effects that different foods were having on me. I saw consistent effects from particular foods. When I moved back to the hubbub of the city for a time, I found that its myriad activities and sensory onslaughts submerged this newfound awareness.

What sort of effects had I noticed? I found that if I had certain foods for breakfast and then worked at home, I would be lethargic all morning and would have to struggle against the temptation to crawl back into bed. On the other hand, I discovered foods that made me feel sharp even while working at home with the silence and the nearby inviting bed. I also noticed that some foods aided me in my editorial work, while others seemed to turn me toward nature to watch the busy woods animals outside.

When I was with people or in my office the numerous tasks and diversions generally overrode the effects of food.

Puzzled but curious about my observations, I began to seek information about the effects of food on mood and behavior. For years I had kept files on the subject, but it hadn't really come together until I began noticing changes in myself. I knew that we are chemical creatures eating chemical foods, but I wondered just which chemicals were involved.

The medical literature on the subject was sparse. Popular books were usually confusing and contradictory. Even when I agreed with a particular author's statements, I rarely discovered an explanation that I could accept scientifically.

Paracelsus, a noted maverick physician of the sixteenth century, made this forceful comment: "The universities do not teach us everything. A good physician should be ready to learn from mid-wives, gypsies, nomads, brigands, people outside the law. He should inquire among all classes of people seeking out everything which might contribute to his knowledge. He should travel widely, undergo many adventures and learn all the while."

So wherever I went, from New York to Big Sur, from Paris to Tokyo, and so many places in between, I asked about foods and studied whatever I could find. I sought out information from diverse sources—restaurateurs, waitresses, witch doctors, herbalists. I delved into anthropology and the history of foods and herbs. I spoke with drug addicts and drug experts (sometimes the same people).

My medical education was woefully deficient when it came to foods. Certainly I had learned some nutrition, but the concepts of food effects were rarely even hinted at in my curriculum.

I realized a basic principle on which this book is based: all foods are chemical compounds. The terms "drug" and "food" are often vague, applied to a substance according to the manner in which it is eaten and how it looks. Protein in a steak is a drug or medicine, as is protein in a capsule.

As my research notes expanded I began to feel that I

should communicate my finds to a wide audience. In addition to the well over a thousand food additives (that may alter behavior), foods exert effects that can shape personalities. Foods can also induce different types of consciousness. With a diet predominated by a certain type of food (e.g., sleep-inducing), effects tend to be cumulative. I began to see implications for food effects in therapies and life adaptations.

People can choose a virtually limitless variety of foods to enhance a desired state. Certainly a person needing to be alert should avoid sleep-inducing substances. On the other hand, a person may be puzzled by his insomnia if he has taken stimulant foods. There are foods conducive to mystical experiences, others to more worldly pursuits. Using this sort of knowledge, we can assist "the wisdom of the body."

Over the years I collected information about chemicals in foods. My files bulged with thousands of pieces of data. Within six months of my joining the faculty of a medical school, interest in this subject had surfaced. I was asked to teach graduate biochemistry courses, was a guest lecturer at undergraduate biology courses, began a medical school elective, and was asked to present a lecture to the department of internal medicine. I was the speaker at "grand rounds" in one department and was asked to expand on the subject of the effects of food on behavior in three additional sessions. Like a mini-avalanche, requests for more information on my "personal" topic began coming in. A major scientific journal expressed interest in a feature article. As all this was occurring I began to enlarge my research, and asked hundreds of students to list the foods and effects they had noticed. I began an undergraduate honors seminar with a laboratory format—the lab being a kitchen where we could prepare and test different meals. In a more social vein, I gave parties that were carefully planned to make maximum use of food power. The practical effects were gratifying.

This perspective on food is based on the most current

research, and many of the findings are at the frontier of the field. One of the leading researchers in the field predicted at a conference in 1978 that in the future people would be able to modify behavior through food. I believe that the "future" he spoke of can actually begin now.

Our scientific knowledge is far from complete. And because we are each unique, our physical and behavioral reactions vary greatly. We are at a frontier, and as with the frontiers of the wilderness there is much land to be cleared. There will be some dead-end trails and some that will lead to fertile territory. As my research continues, I am sure I will find out much more to deepen and extend these concepts. But it is a beginning.

This book was written so that people can begin to understand food power and use this knowledge to enrich their lives.

Introduction: Food Power— 1. An Overview

Every living creature must eat. From the tiny amoeba to the giant whale the common element is the search for food. The movement of prehistoric man was largely governed by his search for food, and the growth of civilization can be traced according to the development of agriculture. When survival is the question, any food becomes the answer; but as foods became more plentiful, their ability to influence behavior and mood became more apparent. The "spice of life" is more than just enhancement of taste.

Centuries ago, explorers set out not for adventure only, but also in search of spices. Columbus discovered a new hemisphere, but all he was looking for was a different route to the Spice Islands. Five years after Columbus's voyage, Vasco da Gama sailed around Africa's Cape of Good Hope to get to the spices of India. So important was his quest that he and his men risked turning black—a superstition current in those times. When he finally returned to Portugal, his cargo of spices was worth more than sixty times what it cost to outfit the expedition. The science of navigation was spurred by the search for food and spices; Magellan's round-the-world voyage, which began in 1519, was paid for by the spices his ships brought back.

Why were spices so valuable? Was it simply for taste enhancement? It was for that and very likely more. People were searching for spices with chemical effects. Pepper, a stimulant and slight euphoriant, was sought. Nutmeg, a stimulant at low doses, produces hallucinations when two cloves are eaten. Ginger root, which has stimulant effects, has been used as a drug in veterinary medicine.

Foods have chemical effects far beyond supplying energy. Some act as strong drugs, others have weaker effects; but taken together in a diet, foods help shape entire personalities. Some foods act as antidepressants, some help induce sleep, some stimulate creativity, some induce mystical states of consciousness. It is even likely that the behavior patterns we call a "national character" are partially brought about by the food choices in a particular region.

If a person takes a drug that affects his mood and behavior, his personality will eventually change. The drug effects of foods—even common, off-the-shelf varieties—similarly modify the personality. The effects don't arise from any additive, but from the natural chemical makeup of the food.

We can readily see some gross effects of powerful foods. For example, the cannabis plant (marijuana) is a vegetable containing calories, vitamins, and minerals; it also has powerful effects on the mind. The coca plant, from which we extract cocaine, is also a good source of vitamins and calories, and also has strong effects. The Peruvian Indians chew the coca leaf almost continually for its stimulant effects which enhance their ability to work at high altitudes. When the Spaniards came to South America they tried to take the coca plant from the Indians, who rebelled and wouldn't work without it.

The psilocybin mushroom contains all the nutritional benefits of a regular mushroom, but has hallucinogenic effects. This so-called magic mushroom is so powerful that the Mexican Aztec Indians felt that a god dwelled within it.

Another powerful food is the peyote cactus, a humble-looking, scrubby plant containing not only calories, vitamins, proteins, minerals, and carbohydrates, but also mescaline, which can induce a markedly altered state of consciousness. In fact, after eating the cactus Aldous Huxley was so impressed that he wrote *The Doors of Perception,* a work celebrating the new insights and enhanced perceptions he had experienced. Many other scholars were similarly excited by their observations; Havelock Ellis, the noted psychologist, urged his friends to try peyote.

Marijuana, psilocybin mushrooms, and peyote cactus are powerful changers of mood, behavior, and perception. You may say, "But those are not foods, they are drugs." Yes, they may well be called drugs, but let us take another perspective.

Imagine a spectrum of foods represented by a horizontal line (Figure 1). At one end of this line are foods that have such powerful effects when taken in small dosages that we call them drugs. At some point along the line we make an arbitrary dividing line—on one side of the dividing line the foods are "drugs," and on the other side the foods are "foods." They are all made of chemicals, but the "foods" are not as powerful in their effects.

SPECTRUM OF FOODS

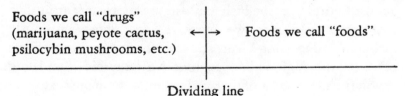

Foods we call "drugs"
(marijuana, peyote cactus,   ←|→   Foods we call "foods"
psilocybin mushrooms, etc.)

Dividing line

Figure 1

Many times it is a question of amount eaten. For example, one or two psilocybin mushrooms may exert powerful effects, but usually we need two or three cups of coffee to feel coffee power. There are many foods in frequent use that can act as strong drugs, but we limit the quantities we take. Two cloves of nutmeg will induce hallucinations because the spice contains the chemical myristin. A small amount of nutmeg sprinkled on eggnog, however, is a stimulant, dilating the eyes and producing a merry state (probably why it is used at Christmastime). Lettuce leaves contain a substance called lactucin, which exerts a calming, slightly euphoric state. But you have to eat a head or two of lettuce to really notice the effects. Lettuce flakes, however, have been put into a cigarette which, according to tests by the magazine *High Times*, clearly has strong effects. Aged cheese contains tyramine which stimulates as do amphetamines and cocaine. In small doses the effects are pleasant, probably accounting for the custom of serving aged cheese at the outset of a party to enliven the guests and get them to be outgoing and talkative.

A consistent diet of a particular food with relatively weak chemical action can have additive effects. For example, the Japanese fish fugu is a potent stimulator of the glands and is a true aphrodisiac. The time-honored claim that seafood stimulates sexuality was expressed in the seventeenth century by Dr. Nicholas Venette in *Tableau de l'Amour.* He wrote, "We have observed in France that those who live almost entirely on shellfish and fish are more ardent in love than others. In fact, we ourselves feel most amorously inclined during Lent." The scientific basis for these effects rests on the high iodine content with thyroid-stimulating action (small amounts of thyroid hormone stimulate sexuality) and the findings of sex-hormonelike chemicals in shellfish, particularly oysters. The important point here is that while a single food might do relatively little, a consistent diet can exert cumulative effects.

Various cultures have recognized the power of foods and have developed diets for special purposes. Knowledge of the chemistry of foods sheds new light on the effectiveness of such diets and allows more respect and appreciation for the wisdom of the ancients. For example, the spare diet or fasting of religious retreats tends to induce a more mystical state of mind. Fasting alters the body metabolism substantially, affecting the brain. The pomegranate, often mentioned in religious works, is a fruit with the chemical pelleterine. Its chemical similarity to mescaline lends some support to Buddha's wisdom, "Eat of the pomegranate. It will cleanse your soul of hatred and envy." The book of the mystical Jewish tradition, the kabbala, has interpreted the "orchard of pomegranates" in the Bible to symbolize religious spirit or souls.

Some religious groups have gone beyond using foods for subtle alterations and use foods of great power in their rituals. The Native American Church of North America uses peyote cactus as part of its ritual, and some Indians in Mexico use psilocybin mushrooms as part of their rites. Are these wild drug parties? Hardly, because the powerful vegetables are deeply embedded in religious traditions and are used to achieve the mystical and visionary state detailed throughout history. This state has been called "cosmic consciousness" and whether naturally induced or aided by a power food, the descriptions of it are remarkably similar. Saint Paul, on the road to Damascus, describes "the revelation of exceeding greatness." Buddha spoke of ". . . passing beyond phenomena, cause him to become an inheritor of the highest heavens, make him one to become multiple; being multiple to become one, and endow him with clear and heavenly vision surpassing that of men." Walt Whitman found, "I am satisfied. I see, dance, laugh, sing, wandering amazed at my own lightness and glee."

Albert Hoffman, a renowned chemist who discovered LSD and extracted and synthesized the active ingredients from the peyote cactus and the psilocybin mushroom, believes that these plants stimulate some religious center in man. Knowing about drug effects of foods and the complexity of the brain, we can view such foods as affecting us chemically rather than as the Aztecs did, worshiping the plants because they believed a god resided in them.

Compare a spare religious diet with the kind of feast that characterized a Roman orgy. Such a feast featured a wide variety of seafood, spicy sausages and meat, milk, eggs, olive oil—all in such large quantities that some nobles needed to regurgitate after each course. The high protein content, the gland-stimulating actions of many of the foods, and the intense oral interests all combined with the setting to stimulate sensuality. The many spices, including salt, pepper, nutmeg, and ginger, added to the stimulation.

Whenever a national or religious group has, so to speak, canonized a particular diet for a particular occasion, the nature of the diet often aids substantially in inducing the mood of the occasion. For example, Yom Kippur, the Jewish Day of Atonement, is the most serious holy day of the year. Observers are required to fast for the entire day, and apart from the aspect of hunger, the absence of food induces a calmer, more introspective mood. On the other hand, the use of stimulant herbs and spices is associated with a holiday of gaiety and merriment like Christmas. The American tradition of Thanksgiving would not be complete without a turkey, which contains a large amount of the amino acid tryptophan. Tryptophan tends to induce sleep; the traditional Thanksgiving dinner ends with people feeling the kind of lethargy that can result from tryptophan. Other components of the Thanksgiving dinner also tend to induce these feelings. The yam may have hormonal actions leading to retention of salt, resulting in a somewhat bloated feeling.

Our bodies are marvelous chemical storehouses in which thousands of chemical reactions occur simultaneously. People used to joke that the components of the human body were worth only a dollar. How untrue. We are all at least "Six Million Dollar" men and women. Hormones, for example, cost as much as $200,000 per gram. Adding up the known hormones and enzymes in our bodies and putting them at current market prices, we see that even $6 million is a low estimate. The point is that since we are made of many chemicals, the foods we take in—apart from their fat, protein, and carbohydrate contents, and their vitamin and mineral effects—can, with their natural chemicals, substantially influence our mental state.

When Eve offered Adam the apple she realized the potent effects of food. Whether the fruit was indeed an apple as we know it is questionable, since the effects were profound. Perhaps it was a thorn apple (also called jimson weed, or the devil's apple), which contains a hallucinogenic chemical. The Koran suggests it was a type of banana. Regardless, plant and food power have been recognized from earliest recorded history.

Physicians of long ago were more concerned with the profound effects of foods than are those of today. Hippocrates, the great Greek physician of the fifth century B.C. who is known as the "Father of Medicine," insisted that diet was the foundation of healing. Few of today's medical schools follow this wisdom.

Diet can powerfully influence our mental states. Choosing a diet for its effects can truly be termed "creative eating." For example, a person who has been having a great deal of difficulty sleeping might find part of the problem to be a diet

with an excess of stimulant-type foods and only a modicum
of foods that tend to induce sleep. Change of diet might
avoid getting into a sleeping pill habit. On the other hand,
a person who finds himself depressed and lethargic might
well find that his diet is overbalanced in terms of sleep-
inducing chemicals. This question must be prominent: Is the
diet at cross-purposes with the individual's life? A religious
diet is at odds with a need for much bodily activity. A diet
to aid in sleeping is at odds with a lively or creative life.

Let's take an illustrative case. A 38-year-old woman has
a feeling of lethargy and low energy. She has what appears to
be normal problems of living but no serious stresses. Her
diet is as follows:

BREAKFAST	LUNCH	DINNER
1 poppy seed roll	Lettuce salad with	Turkey with
2 eggs	radishes and cut	seasonings
1 glass of milk	cabbage	Carrots
1 cup of valerian	1 banana	Peas
tea		1 baked potato
		Pineapple
		1 glass of
		Burgundy wine

What about this diet might be related to her general
feelings of lethargy? The breakfast contains poppy seeds,
some of which have a low opium content. The eggs are high
in choline, which tends to be calming, and, in fact, choline
can precipitate depression in sensitive people. The milk, with
its concentration of tryptophan, stimulates sleepiness. The
valerian tea has actually been used to induce sleep.

At lunch, the salad has lactucin from the lettuce, which
is slightly calming. The radishes and cabbage have mild
antithyroid actions due to the presence of thiouracil which,
in concentrated form, is used as a drug to control overactive
thyroids. The banana contains sleep-inducing tryptophan.

The dinner meat is the highest in tryptophan, and the monosodium glutamate seasoning makes many people sleepy. The carrots have mild salt-retaining effects and the peas contain a chemical with mildly antithyroid actions. The potato tends to induce drowsiness. The pineapple is high in tryptophan, and the Burgundy wine is a depressant.

This woman's diet has a preponderance of foods that induce sleep, increase fluid retention, and mildly depress the thyroid. If followed for days and weeks it can cumulatively shape her behavior. Change of diet might not have much effect if she has a significant depression—which is a biochemical phenomenon—but before drugs and psychotherapy, dietary change might be worthwhile. If she is being treated with medicines or psychiatric intervention, this diet is working against change.

Let's take another example of how food power can work against us. A 45-year-old man has been treated for high blood pressure for one year. He has needed a great deal of medication that causes depression and sexual problems. Yet his blood pressure is still high and he is getting more and more worried. We look at his diet and find:

BREAKFAST	LUNCH	DINNER
2 cups of coffee	Pickled herring	Aged cheese with
1 ripe banana	Chicken livers in	crackers
1 cup of yogurt	sour cream sauce	Chinese rice and
	Chocolate mousse	soy sauce
	1 beer	Salt and pepper
		1 glass of sherry

As his doctor advised him, this man is not eating much; but let's look at what he is eating. For breakfast, the coffee is a stimulant that raises blood pressure; the ripe banana and the yogurt contain tyramine, which also acts to elevate the pressure. At lunch, the pickled herring has tyramine as do the chicken livers, sour cream, and beer. The chocolate is a stimulant. At dinner, both the aged cheese and the soy sauce contain pressure-elevating tyramine. The sherry also contains a small amount of tyramine. So what we find is a man who is on such a stimulating diet that his blood pressure is sky-high, he has severe headaches, and his medication can't keep up with what he is eating. Before even starting potent pressure-lowering medication with its many many side effects, he should have tried a low blood pressure diet. Knowledge of food power might save this man's life.

What about social events and parties? Parties bring special joys to life by bringing people together. But people are different and hostesses and hosts give different kinds of parties; the foods served should be chosen to enhance the mood of the gathering—not be at cross-purposes. Some foods (as well as settings) are well suited to entertaining business associates. A religious gathering might well require a different menu than a gathering of old and intimate friends. In chapter 12, a variety of party foods will be described, and sample situations, menus, and settings will be suggested.

Reader beware! Look at labels and ingredients! Chocolate, for example, contains enlivening substances that stimulate talk and enhance pleasurable moods—but many supposed chocolate-containing foods do not involve real chocolate at all, or have only a small amount. It was a shock when I discovered the truth about my favorite "chocolate" candy bars.

The processing of foods may produce some variations. For example, the tyramine in aged cheese, mentioned earlier, is not found in the processed products even though the taste might be similar. It is the aging process that converts the amino acid tyrosine into the stimulating amine tyramine.

Compound effects must be avoided. For example, Chianti wine contains tyramine and serving it with aged cheese gives many people headaches. On the other hand, serving aged cheese with a strong sedative wine (such as Burgundy) will offset the stimulation. All wines do not have tranquilizing action. There are stimulant wines, wines for relaxation, and some good for sleep.

Sections in libraries and bookstores with books about food are expanding rapidly, but with few exceptions the advice given is based on folklore, tradition, "Grandmother's wisdom," and occasionally a dash of scientific information. Some is accurate, but which? The dilemma is similar to one posed by my professor of medicine. He said, "Based on the changes which have occurred in the past fifty years, half of what I tell you will prove to be either misleading or false. The problem is which half?" He implored the class to always ask the question "Why?" In this book, "why" will be answered wherever possible.

Chicken soup is indeed good for a cold. Why? It is good not simply because Grandmother says it is (although Grandma's wisdom is often precise and correct) or because a food expert says it is. When properly prepared with suitable chicken and other ingredients, the chemical makeup includes components found in "cold medicines" as well as substances known to stimulate body reactions that diminish cold symptoms and strengthen immune responses, or defenses against colds.

If I say a particular food is good for your spleen, you might or might not believe it. You might accept it on faith because of your trust in my medical degree, or you might reject it for the very same reason—many people feel physicians by and large are not food experts. In either case you could not easily verify what I say. How does a person know if his spleen is working better? Perhaps there are a few sensitive people who are aware of the state of their internal organs; nervous impulses arise from body organs and go to the brain, but these are not usually perceived consciously.

The overwhelming majority of people cannot test for themselves whether an herb, spice, plant, or other food is benefiting their livers or spleens. But the brain is a responding organ that makes us aware of our moods, our feelings of energy or lethargy, our creative powers, our sexual interests, the tone of our parties.

The chemical composition of the foods discussed will be described whenever possible in the following pages. Many years of research have gone into this study of the chemistry of food. The overall concept of using foods for a purpose is a new way to view foods. The lock-step nutritional evaluations where certain vitamins, fats, proteins, and carbohydrates are measured represent only a portion of the effects food have upon us.

Many common foods have not undergone chemical analysis. Some analyses are outdated because processing techniques can alter the chemical nature of foods. For example, pasteurization of juices markedly changes vitamin and chemical makeup. Storage produces change, as does freezing and drying. With more knowledge of chemical contents, however, we can more clearly understand foods and their effects. As we learn more we can avoid the "seat of the pants flying" that goes into so many diets. Nutritionists generally concern themselves with known nutrients in food rather than with the other chemicals and their drug effects. Food as therapy for mental states is only in the first stages of experimentation.

Some nutritionists will be puzzled by this book. One has already asked me what the chemical composition of foods has to do with nutrition if the chemicals are not any of the known nutrients. A good question. First, many of the chemicals may well act in a similar fashion as vitamins, but there has been virtually no research in depth in this area. Also, the chemicals may be extremely powerful in shaping our mental state but have no known role in nutrition per se, although their effects on the metabolism of the cell are profound. For example, the stimulant caffeine from coffee, nutmeg with its myristin, the gingerol in ginger root have no known role in the traditional nutritional sense—but few would argue that they have powerful effects.

Some drug-oriented people will extract from this book only information about foods with strong drug effects. Such thrill-seeking is not uncommon, but it is a terribly narrow view. Creative eating means using food to help induce particular states of mind, counter undesirable states of mind or feelings, and to help us find balance.

The concept of a balanced diet is important. Excesses in anything are rarely healthy. Understanding that a particular food is a stimulant can help us to balance. Remember, a person can overdose on a food just as he or she might overdose on a drug. If one portion of a particular food is helpful, it is far from correct to think that three helpings will be three times as good.

In the next chapter we will look at the effects of ordinary foods—not from a health food store or some far-out head shop, but right at the supermarket.

2 ⌁ At the Supermarket

It's shopping day and we're off to the market. Let's start at the vegetable counter. First we see good leafy lettuce, a member of the genus *Lactuca*. It contains small amounts of lactucin, a chemical that produces relaxation when a good amount is taken. Lettuce extract and the dried juices from wild lettuce (*Lactuca virosa*) is termed "lettuce opium," and will induce a marijuanalike sensation when smoked or eaten. An additional active component of the same lettuce is hyoscyamine, which is present in very small quantities. Hyoscyamine is similar to the medicine scopolamine, previously in widespread use in obstetrics to induce twilight sleep.

Next to the lettuce there is a luxurious bunch of celery. The Greeks used to give celery as a prize to victorious athletes; physicians have used the stimulant and diuretic (water-losing) properties of the celery seed for centuries, particularly for menstrual discomfort.

Near the celery we find carrots. In addition to having a high level of vitamin A, carrots and carrot seeds also exert estrogen (a female hormone) actions. *The New York Times* in 1975 reported on a village where heavy ingestion of carrots and carrot seeds had caused a decreased birth rate owing to effects like those of birth control pills.

As we continue, we see some nice Idaho potatoes which should be good eating. However, if any of the green leaves or stems of the plant are around, they will contain some potent alkaloids. The potato is a member of the deadly nightshade family and the leaves contain belladonna-type compounds used in scopolamine. In small doses these leaves will produce a very dry mouth and drowsiness; in larger dosages, hallucinations; in still larger doses, they can be fatal. This is the reason potato leaves are carefully removed. The leaves also contain steroidlike substances and glycosides, chemicals similar to the digitalis doctors prescribe for heart patients. The dangerous character of the leaves led to an intense, fifty-year debate in eighteenth-century France over whether potatoes were safe to eat and whether restrictions were to be placed on importations. Small green potatoes may contain appreciable amounts of toxic substances, accounting for the twenty deaths from potato poisoning reported in medical literature. Edible potatoes still have small amounts of alkaloids that cause drowsiness in sensitive people.

Beautiful red tomatoes now come into our view. The tomato fruit itself is tasty and rich in vitamin C, but the green leaves and stems contain substances similar to those found in potato leaves. The roots and leaves contain a complex chemical substance called tomatine, also found in the fruit in very low concentration. Tryptamine, present in low concentration, can cause hallucinations if you eat a lot of tomatoes. Artificially ripened tomatoes probably have altered chemical constituents, but comparative testing hasn't been done.

The artificial ripening process deserves some explanation. Ordinarily, a garden tomato will be firm and green along its gradual path to ripeness. Often tomatoes are picked while still green because they are firmer and ship better. They are then exposed to high concentrations of ethylene gas, which rapidly turns the outer skin bright red and gives a semblance of ripeness. But the insides haven't ripened on the vine— this accounts for the relatively tasteless tomatoes often found on supermarket shelves.

Now the mushrooms. These are pretty bland; later, as we take a field trip, we can find mushrooms with "magic." Almost all mushrooms sold in the United States are field mushrooms (*Agericus campestris*), which are mild in taste and chemical effect.

Here is a little spearmint. It contains some compounds with mild stimulant action. Its principal chemical, carvone, is also found in caraway seeds.

Many vegetables such as kale, broccoli, cabbage, and turnips have a mild antithyroid effect, as do soybeans, mustard seed, and horseradish. Because the thyroid gland is involved with metabolism, a diet consistently overbalanced with such foods could result in slight energy-depressant actions.

Garlic is thought by gypsies to exert beneficial effects even when a clove is simply worn about the neck. This potent vegetable contains antibioticlike substances and carries a reputation of being a tonic, clearing lungs and brain, and strengthening breathing. It acts on parasites in the intestine, thereby aiding health and general feelings of well-being.

What about sprouts? There are some alfalfa sprouts and barley sprouts containing hordenine, a compound which acts as a mild stimulant. It is similar in structure to amphetamine and to tyramine, the stimulant found in aged cheese.

Hops! This is an unusual store. I thought we'd have to wait until the beer section, but we're in luck. A soup made with hops (the flowering tops of *Humulus lupulus*) gets you jolly and tranquil, but men beware! It also has some estrogen effects.

Parsley is a source of apiol, which produces some sedation and keeps a fever down. It has been made into a tea or smoked for its sedative effects, as has sage. Sage also has been used to aid irregular menstrual flow.

The next stop on our trip is the fruit section. A shipment of tropical fruits has arrived. The pomegranate catches our eye. This is a complex fruit containing alkaloids mostly of the pelleterine variety, similar to the sedative tryptophan and tryptamine. Both of these are part of the serotonin system in brain chemistry, which is thought to have a lot to do with tranquility and involve the "third eye" of intuition. The pomegranate is also a source of female hormones. One biochemist has pointed out that the anise fruit, the pomegranate, and the palm kernel all have natural estrogen effects which might result in some antifertility tendencies as well as some personality changes.

Next, there are mangoes. Andrew Weil, author of *The Natural Mind* and one of the country's leading drug experts, said, "I don't know whether it's possible to convey the joy of my discovery of mangoes." Let's look at the mangoes offered for sale here. If they are hard, seek further because for the real mango experience you have to have one that's been sun-ripened in the climate where it was grown—that leads to the greatest juiciness. Ripe mangoes stimulated Paramahansa Yogananda to comment in *Autobiography of a Yogi*, "It is impossible for the Hindu to conceive of a heaven without mangoes." The anacardic acid and anacardiol found in mangoes bear familial resemblances to drugs used to treat depression.

Now for some luscious cherries. Beware of the stems and pits, which may be toxic. They are similar to apricot pits, which are the base for the controversial drug laetrile.

Strawberries contain a chemical that causes tranquility. Artificial strawberry flavor lacks this—an example of technology removing a good food/drug.

Moving on, there are some fine ripe watermelons. They

have some chemicals that increase urinary flow, but in addition contain a complicated chemical called cucurbocitrin which lowers blood pressure and exerts a calming effect. Perhaps the image of eating a watermelon on a lazy afternoon has a sounder scientific basis than most people think.

As we push our cart onward we find a real treat—one of the earliest known fruits from the Fertile Crescent, the fig. Called the most natural source of sugar, it contains the simplest sugar, glucose, which is used for energy by the brain, along with the calming amino acid tryptophan. Dates share this tranquilizing property. For the higher consciousness, Buddha advised a diet of figs, nuts, and dates.

At the end of the fruit counter is a yellow profusion of bananas. Bananas contain tryptophan, an amino acid that is a sleep inducer and a source of tranquility, and that may have antidepressant qualities. The banana is a complex fruit containing many other chemicals. Is there something to the expression "going bananas"? A few years ago there was talk about smoking banana skins for special effects. Some banana skins do contain bufotenine, which can produce hallucinations. Bufotenine is also found in some mushrooms and in toad skin, a frequent component of legendary witches' brews.

What about "going nuts"? Protein is an important component of most nuts; there is also a relatively high tryptophan content. Tryptophan is involved in the synthesis of serotonin, which is found in the pineal gland. This gland is actually a third eye in some reptiles, but in man it is a tiny structure within the brain. Mystics feel it is our "third eye" or "the mind's eye," and it is associated with wisdom and "seeing the light." The peanut is a good source of tryptophan; a diet high in peanuts might tend to induce more serotonin production and, perhaps, a predisposition toward religion.

The kola nut is the source of a variety of alkaloids including caffeine. Sometimes it can be found in nut stores or gourmet supermarkets. The areca nut (or betel nut) is rarely found in America, but in some cultures it is chewed throughout the day for its calming effects owing to the alkaloid arecoline. The cashew nut (an unlikely relative of the mango) contains anacordic acid and anacardiol—the latter has seen medical use as an analeptic (invigorator).

The next stop on our supermarket trip is the herb counter. Among the gifts brought to the Christ Child were frankincense and myrrh. Myrrh contains some pleasantly stimulating actions and has been prized throughout history as a preservative.

Borage is hard to find, but Roger Bacon said that it "maketh the English sprightly." Saffron, from the crocus, has definite stimulant effects. Christopher Catton, an eighteenth-century Englishman, wrote of saffron, "the virtue thereof pierceth to the heart, provoking laughter and merriment."

Valerian is an herb used for thousands of years as a sedative. In fact, Dr. A. Manson, in an article in the *British Medical Journal* in 1928, termed valerian "the earliest method of treating the neuroses"; it was widely used after World War I to treat shell shock. In his classic book, *Therapeutics and Materia Medica,* Dr. Alfred Stillé, professor of medicine at the University of Pennsylvania in 1874, had this to say about valerian: "Nothing is more astonishing in the operation of remedies than the promptness and certainty with which a dose of valerian dispells the gloomy vision of the hypochondriac, calms the hurry and agitation of nervous excitement, allays commencing spasm and diffuses a soothing calm over the whole being of one who but an hour before was prey to a thousand morbid sensations and thick-coming fancies of danger, wrong or loss."

Nutmeg is a spacy spice which in small doses can result in hallucinations. The active element is myristin and the effects can be similar to those seen with LSD and mescaline.

Pepper also contains small amounts of myristin as well

as a stimulant known as piperine. The pepper must be freshly ground, however, since chemical changes occur, resulting in decreased effect.

Be careful not to get high on your Christmas decorations! Absurd, you say? Not at all. The smoke of Christmas laurel induces strange dreams and visions, and the mistletoe berry is a powerful and dangerous stimulant.

As we continue our supermarket trip we come to the coffee section. The main alkaloid in coffee, caffeine, has a long and exciting history. Tea contains the alkaloid theophylline, a stimulant that is also good for treating colds and clearing the lungs.

On the next counter is a profusion of breads. There is some evidence that in the seventeenth century some rye was infested with the ergot-producing fungus, which may have resulted in bread with LSD-like effects. Even more intriguing, this bread may have accounted for the visions of young girls and subsequent cries of witchcraft by the townspeople. However, the ergot fungus is now well controlled and we won't find it in bread. So we find an attractive loaf of bread covered with poppy seeds. According to two pharmacologists at the University of Illinois, there is opium in some of the poppy seeds found on bread and rolls. Eating enough of these poppy seeds will induce opium effects. From opium, by the way, come morphine, codeine, and heroin. What about other breads? Dr. Claude Frazier reported, in 1978, that wheat products can make sensitive people fatigued.

Our next stop is the candy counter. It's getting harder and harder to find real chocolate in candy these days, but there is some. Chocolate is one of those special foods containing a caffeinelike substance called theobromine, which means "food of the gods." (See chapters 6 and 8 for more about chocolate's stimulant and aphrodisiac qualities.) And vanilla has a long medical history as a nervous-system stimulant.

If you can find some real licorice you're in for a special treat. As those who know licorice can attest, there are substances in it that produce a delicious, slightly euphoric state. Overdosage of licorice, unfortunately, has resulted in elevation of blood pressure in some people. For licorice aficionados, it is interesting to note that there are more than a hundred different varieties of licorice in the world, and that this ancient candy was used in Chinese religious ceremonies thousands of years ago. Pieces of licorice root were even found in King Tut's tomb. Alas, much of the licorice sold in supermarkets is synthetic.

Before going on to the meat counter, a review of our brief supermarket tour might be useful. There are some caveats that a careful food shopper should know. First, most of the time we use spices in such small amounts that most people can't detect any chemical action. Exceptions are mace, nutmeg, and possibly freshly ground pepper. Monosodium glutamate is used in abundance, and the effects of sleepiness, headache, and sweating have been noted in medical literature as the Chinese Restaurant Syndrome. These effects are usually thought to be transient, but this may not always be true. A University of California psychiatrist wrote in the *New England Journal of Medicine* in October 1978 that his wife and nine-year-old son apparently experienced psychiatric disorders due to MSG. In fact, he reported that his wife underwent a two-week depressive syndrome which was thought to be caused by monosodium glutamate. Once this was suspected, his wife was given a test dose of a bowl of wonton soup, and she had an immediate reaction and another depression which lasted two weeks.

It is important to understand the balancing nature of foods. There is nothing wrong with eating soybeans, for example, even though they contain a compound that is antithyroid. What is wrong is eating a food excessively or as too great a percentage of the diet. If a person has a problem such as an abnormally low thyroid function, he should attempt to reduce the intake of those foods that tend to aggravate the condition.

Yams can have some estrogen effects—in fact, a factory has been established to produce estrogen from yams. If the yam becomes more than 25 percent of a man's diet, he might have some problems. However, there is not a shred of evidence that eating a moderate amount of yams causes any problem at all. But, if a man is having some problems with diminished libido, he should reduce quantities of foods that might exert estrogen effects. On the other hand, a woman who is entering menopause or has had a hysterectomy should try to include some foods with estrogen actions in her diet—not to excess, of course.

Now, at the meat counter, we see a bewildering choice of red meats. Since red meat is the muscle of the beef animal, its chemical composition is extremely complex, and includes vitamins, minerals, hormones, enzymes, and any other chemicals that might have been fed to the animal close to the day of slaughter. A pound of most beef contains two to four grams of the amino acid tryptophan. Since only one to two grams of tryptophan is sufficient to induce sleep in most people, it is easy to understand why many people find that a large meat meal makes them feel drowsy.

In my research, of some fifty people who volunteered the information that red meat had an effect on them, only two felt that a meat meal gave them energy. The other comments were couched in such words as "drowsy," "lethargic," "sedentary," "heavy," "full," "melancholy," "depressed," and "sluggish." One person felt "contented" after a meat meal and another said meat gave her a feeling of "safety and security." With regard to other meats, most felt that pork had less of an effect than beef. Lamb chops were felt by most to have less soporific effects, and all felt that chicken had the least effect in terms of feeling sleepy or sluggish.

There has been no comparative analysis of chemical

content other than protein content in various cuts of meat. Of some interest is that the better the cut, the more fat present. But in terms of behavioral effects, meats have not been analyzed with food power in mind. The location of a particular cut, however, may lead one to suspect that it has a richer nutritional content. The filet mignon is an internal muscle in the back of the abdominal cavity. It is at a consistently higher temperature during life than muscles in the rump, extremities, or more superficial areas. Also, it is bathed by a better blood supply because of its location.

Of all fowl, turkey meat has the greatest percentage of the amino acid tryptophan. Perhaps the feeling of lethargy after the Thanksgiving turkey directly reflects this fact.

Chicken used to have a better reputation. Chickens are maintained in houses where they have little room to move about—a condition that blunts an animal's glandular responses. In times past a chicken was killed by cutting off its head, which led to a wild, thrashing chicken and hence the phrase "running around like a chicken without a head." The effect of this kind of slaughter is to have a clear airway for a great release of the inhibitory controls upon the chicken's glands. As a result the chicken is actually working with all glands on full speed—the chicken meat is supercharged. Many chickens are now commercially slaughtered by suffocation after an electric shock is administered to their head. As a result, during the last few minutes of life, toxins and waste products are building up.

Parts of the chicken may provide some beneficial effects. A stock made by simmering chicken hearts and adrenal glands will contain adrenalinelike substances. Only the hearts and adrenals should be used for optimum results. Stock made by simmering the testes will contain hormone building blocks. Ideally, there could be a "male soup" and a "female soup," with the male organs and the hearts in the "male" and the ovaries, adrenal glands, and kidneys in the "female."

Chicken livers are considered by many to be a delicacy and, in fact, their tyramine content may make them a stimulating dish.

Many anthropologists believe that our meat-eating habits are quite different from what they were during our early evolution. For one thing, hunting was done during particular seasons. If the hunting was good in the fall, people ate meat then and in the winter (since the cold would preserve the kill). In the springtime and summer there would be little meat. Our bodies would naturally store a surplus for the times when the hunt wasn't so good. There would then be periods of feast and relative famine. Meat-eating all year long is a phenomenon of our technological society, and results in a tendency toward obesity and possibly heart disease and stroke.

Before heading for the checkout counter we should stop by the beverage section. Many beverages were much stronger in terms of their druglike actions in the past. For example, Coca-Cola was originally made with cocaine and kola nut extract; with the powerful stimulant from the coca leaf, along with the caffeinelike substances from the kola nut, this was a strong concoction indeed. After about 1900 cocaine was outlawed and most cola beverages these days have artificially added caffeine. However, Coca-Cola is still made from coca leaves—the cocaine has been extracted, but there are some alkaloids from the coca leaf present. Many people not only can detect the difference between "Coke" and "Pepsi," but insist on drinking the former because of the coca extract. Ginger ale was originally more powerful than it is today because it contained extract from ginger root. Most of it these days is artificially flavored and colored.

If you open a book about food that lists nutritional values, how do you apply the information to a particular food you have just bought at a supermarket? The value listed might be completely inaccurate! For example, what happens if you analyze fruits and leafy vegetables for ascorbic acid (vitamin C) content, knowing their different growth conditions? Light affects vitamin C content markedly. The vitamin C content of turnip greens can be raised almost ten times by exposure to more light. Tomato plants grown in the sun have twice the vitamin C of those grown in the shade, even though the fruit does not look much different. In one experiment tomatoes were stored in the dark overnight, which led to a marked reduction in ascorbic acid content.

What about vitamin A? There is substantially less in tomatoes that mature in the dark than those that mature in the light. There is also less in hothouse tomatoes. Thiamine (vitamin B_1) is also increased when fruit matures in the light.

Understanding the powerful effects of sunlight allows us to gauge vitamin content and amounts of other chemical constituents. What about tomatoes that are harvested when green because they are firmer and ship better, and then are exposed in a gas chamber to ethylene chloride which produces a rapid surface reddening? How are they nutritionally? These tomatoes are likely to be nutritionally inferior to a tomato vine-ripened with plenty of sunshine.

The time of harvest may also be important. One study showed a spring harvest of beans gave higher vitamin B_1 levels than a fall harvest.

Thus, a number indicating nutritional content might be misleading unless the growth conditions are known. Do food producers know this? Many producers are totally unaware of the influences these variables have on chemical content. Others might know, but cannot measure the nutritional value and even if they could, would not wish to suffer the economic hardship of changing their procedures. On the other hand, the consumer must be aware of the importance of growth conditions. One experiment demonstrated that herbivorous animals fed food grown in soil deficient in trace elements developed malnutrition. We, like herbivorous animals, are what we eat—or aren't what we are deprived of. If we eat deficient food, we become deficient.

This relates to animal foods as well. Nutritional value may not be at all correlated with the weight of the animal, for example, and marked differences in value can exist in milk, meat, and eggs.

What about fruits? Much depends on where they are grown, how long the fruit is left on the tree, and the time of storage. If taken from the tree too soon, fruit undergoes a premature stoppage of ripening processes.

Storage can be a problem. Stored citrus fruits can lose some ascorbic acid. One study showed that spinach lost 30 percent of its vitamin A content when put in cold storage for five to six days. It lost more than half of its vitamin C content when stored at room temperature for three days.

Processing of various sorts can appreciably alter chemical composition. For example, fruit and vegetable juices are pasteurized to increase stability and shelf life, and to facilitate extraction in some instances. One study on tomato juice showed a loss of one-third the vitamin C and one-third the vitamin A content owing to heating during the canning process. Added to this was loss because of shelf storage.

What about freezing? One analysis showed that frozen asparagus, peas, and lima beans stored at 16°F lost more than 50 percent of their vitamin C in two months; the loss was much less at 0°F.

Then one has to consider ways of cooking and exposure to heat. Foods kept in a steam table at a restaurant often suffer substantial losses of nutrients because of chemical changes from the prolonged steaming.

There has been no large-scale comparative study of commercially grown versus organically grown vegetables in terms of the above factors. Certainly organically grown

vegetables are frequently smaller than those grown commercially, but this may have no bearing on nutritional and
chemical content.

These effects of sunlight, storage, and processing on
vitamins demonstrates how foods may vary. If a food is
expected to have a particular chemical effect, it should be
fresh and unprocessed and, if a fruit, left on the tree or vine
until ripe.

Confronted by these insights about how foods may vary,
is there anything a discerning shopper can do?

The answer is, not a whole lot—if he or she wants to
maintain the vast array of foods in his or her larder. However,
here are some solid suggestions:

1. Buy fruit and vegetables that are grown nearby—they
   will be in season.
2. Read and ask questions about where a particular fruit
   or vegetable comes from, when it was picked, whether
   it was vine-ripened.
3. Sample the fruits and vegetables in different stores.
   Sometimes the difference in taste—which will probably
   reflect growing conditions—will make it obvious that
   one fruit or vegetable is superior.
4. "Bargain" fruits and vegetables that are withered and
   old are rarely true bargains nutritionally.
5. Find out when the store received the shipment and how
   it is being stored. Room-temperature or slightly cooler
   environments are no substitute for a room designed to
   preserve fresh vegetables.
6. Seek a co-op of concerned people who will arrange for
   their own produce shipments. You might not save much
   money, but you will usually be assured of a fresher
   product.
7. Buy fresh fruits and vegetables the day you will be
   using them or the day before. Stockpiling makes life
   easier but is less effective nutritionally.
8. Find out what day each store expects its produce
   delivery. Then plan your shopping to correlate with the
   store that has the most recent shipment.

3 ⌒ Foods for a Purpose

Using food power for a purpose requires some planning and exercise of the intellect. We first must decide what mood or state of consciousness we desire and then determine which foods we need as well as what settings are necessary to make it happen.

"We are what we eat" is by now a tired cliché and it is inaccurate as well. We are *what we eat, where we eat, with whom we eat, how we eat,* and *when we eat.*

First, *what we eat*—we are composed of chemicals synthesized from the basic foodstuffs of our diet. Recent research has shown, for example, that varying levels of the amino acids tryptophan and tyrosine due to fluctuating dietary intake help determine concentration of important amines in the brain that have to do with sleep, depression, and mood. Another major neurotransmitter, acetylcholine, is related to the choline and lecithin in our diet. This sort of linkage illustrates how our mood and behavior are, to an important degree, dependent on what we eat.

Where we eat—different localities have different soil and plant composition; the water, minerals, and trace elements are different. We gradually become closer to our physical environment as our bodies take in the foods of the area.

We are where we eat in another sense. The environment shapes our chemical reactions. Whether we are comfortable in our environment, whether we are in sunshine or shade, whether we are cold or warm—these all affect our body, shifting our metabolism, changing our hormone balances, speeding or slowing intestinal actions and flows of digestive juices. We are creatures responsive to subtle environmental influences.

We are dynamic organisms. The food we take in is varied, and the same food varies in chemical composition from place to place. The Buddhist maxim, "You never step into the same stream twice" is accurate—the water is always moving; our bodies are constantly changing.

With whom we eat—the talk, the social setting, the feelings between people, our comfort or discomfort, whether we are in love or in despair all affect our utilization of food. A wise old woman once told me that when you are in love "you can live on air." Perhaps not entirely on air, but the overall body tone is so high and body efficiency so great that body reactions may be at their best.

Mood affects the digestive processes and with change of mood comes a different rate of nutrient absorption. "The stomach is tied to the mood" is an ancient wisdom that has more scientific force now that the intricate couplings in the nervous system are better understood.

Evidence that social interactions affect eating behavior is widespread, and most people can verify changes in their own behavior. In experiments with monkeys, social isolation resulted in persistent overeating—in fact, twice as much food and liquid was consumed. A persistent stressful environment also resulted in eating more.

How we eat—Are we rushed? Thoughtful? Angry? Happy? All these affect body reactions and digestive processes. Fritz Perls, one of the great Gestalt psychotherapists, once suggested that the act of eating relates to the whole personality; the question "How do you eat?" will therefore form a microcosmic view of the macrocosmic person. For example, a person who eats in a structured manner, with specific mealtimes and a need for a complete meal, lives much of his or her life in just such a structured manner. Conversely, an unstructured person who eats in a hit-or-miss fashion depending on hunger and mood has parallel traits in other activities. Apropos of this, one European traveler in the United States noted the tendency of Americans to bolt down their food on the run and concluded that, in general, America is "a nation of moody dyspeptics."

When we eat—our bodies have their own rhythms of enzyme activity, biochemical reactivity, temperature cycles, and hormonal cycles. At least two hundred of these circadian cycles occur during the day. We generally eat with little thought of the cycles, but they are important. If the metabolism is ready for the food as it is absorbed, our bodies are efficient. If not, we are out of rhythm and the food enters our bodies but is limited in what it can do. "We got rhythm," and understanding this sort of rhythm may be of the utmost importance in maintaining health and in understanding food effects. For example, if it is an active hormone-synthesizing time and the needed proteins, amino acids, etc. are supplied in synchrony, then the efficiency is great. If not, the amino acids and proteins are metabolized in another way, stored, or excreted.

What are some of these rhythms? The rhythm of amino acids in the blood relates to availability of a particular part of a protein enzyme. Due to this cyclical pattern, a meal eaten at 8 A.M. will result in higher amino acid levels than the same meal eaten at 8 P.M.

Our daily body rhythms must be respected, and some are remarkably stubborn to change. One study of watchmen who had worked night shifts for twenty years showed that they all reverted to the traditional sleep-wake pattern when on vacation. There are daily rhythms of hormone secretion, urine formation, enzyme synthesis. Studies on drugs demonstrate that they have more powerful effects when given at particular times.

Certain rhythms are changed only with difficulty. Others can be more easily modified. Our diet produces a rhythm that correlates with our intake of foods. Thus, large shifts and irregular patterns in eating tend to confuse our bodies. Let's say a person was used to having a high-protein breakfast every morning. A rhythm of metabolism would be established, that is, there would be production of certain enzymes to metabolize this food. If one morning there was no breakfast, the rhythm would continue even though there was no food on which to act. If there was total fasting, the rhythm would gradually be reduced. This is why after fasting for more than a few days, it is important to restart food intake slowly.

The complex induction of body enzymes by eating is just beginning to be elucidated, and the beauty and intricacy of the mechanism is astounding. It should cause us to reevaluate all our concepts about diet. The first important step in understanding diet is to see that we are talking about more than just food. Let us think in terms of the whole range and complexity of forces in a balanced diet.

A balanced diet is one that supplies us with all the nutrients we need for our activities at a particular time. A balanced diet for a star athlete preparing for competition is not a balanced diet for a devout person preparing for a religious retreat. Is there a "right" diet? There can't be a right diet for everyone—just a proper diet for a particular person involved in or preparing for a particular activity. The diet should be consistent during that period of time so the body can make good use of the food by adjusting its metabolism. The world demands many actions from us—physical labor, creative thought, religious contemplation, and so on. Fasting can be fine for a religious retreat, dangerous if prolonged physical exertion is needed. Consider the state Milton described in "Il Penseroso":

> And joyn with thee calm Peace, and Quiet,
> Spare Fast, that oft with gods doth diet.

This is hardly the mental state we need for physical exertion.

Nutrition is a great unexplored area in science, medicine, and health. What is adequate? Optimal? One person's adequate or optimal might be another's deficiency state.

Little research has been done in the chemistry of foods. But its importance to us is clear. Understanding food is a major component of twenty-first-century healing.

The myth of the "balanced diet" is in need of exposure. It looks great on a plate—a little bit of this, a little bit of that, all adding up to provide "proper" calories, "proper" vitamins, "proper" minerals—but this is two-dimensional, for it neglects the dynamics of chemical interaction.

The words "balanced diet" are misleading if the interpretation is that each *meal* must have balance. Rather, the *diet* must be balanced over a period of one, two, or three weeks. In fact, a "balanced" meal can cause difficulties due to food interactions. For example, certain vegetables and fruits such as blackberries, beets, red cabbage, and Brussels sprouts act to destroy vitamin B_1 (thiamine). If vitamin B_1 foods such as grains are eaten with these vegetables or fruits, the available thiamine will be reduced.

Foods high in oxalates, such as spinach, chard, beet tops, and rhubarb, act to bind calcium. Thus when milk is taken with them, less calcium is available to the body.

Soybeans contain phytic acid, a chemical that binds zinc. Zinc deficiency has occurred in animals when each feeding included soybean meal.

The point is that the "balanced" meal may involve chemical interactions that render nutrients less available to the body.

Furthermore, the bulk of American food comes highly processed, in brightly colored packages. A recommended balanced diet often involves the known food values of fresh food—not what eventually enters the digestive system of the eater. "Many a slip twixt the cup and the lip" must now be expanded to "Many a change in food value from the harvest to the stomach." As Marshall McLuhan poignantly said, "With increasing sophistication and decreasing understanding, opportunity for ineptitude has greatly increased."

Different cultures have developed systems to understand food and its effects. They saw food power, but did not have the scientific knowledge to explain the effects through chemical-biochemical links. For example, the yoga perspective divided foods into those causing inertia, stimulation, or clarity; the Chinese perspective involved yin and yang foods.

In the Chinese philosophy, the "chi," or wholeness, is composed of yin (female energy—dark, moist, odorous, sleepy) and yang (male principle—intellectual, concentrated, worldly, heat-producing). According to this model, all people have these two principles in varying amounts, and the object is to balance the yin and yang. Over-yin causes health problems to be treated by adding yang and decreasing yin. The converse is also true.

Can these views be reconciled with biochemical understanding? Certainly not entirely, but to some extent sleep-inducing foods generally relate to the yoga inertia foods and Chinese yin foods. Foods that produce insomnia or that are described as "talk foods" are more yanglike or stimulatory. Foods eaten for sexuality are generally inertia or yin foods, while those for religious and creative states tend toward clarity and are more yanglike.

4 ⬎ Foods and Moods

The charts that comprise this chapter should be read with two points in mind.

The first concerns what statisticians call the bell-shaped curve, which is familiar to all students who have labored through a statistics course. What the bell-shaped curve actually shows is that we are all different in our responses. Consider a cup of coffee. Some people are sensitive to its effects and complain of shakiness even before they are finished with a single cup. Others feel that way after one, two, or even three cups. And then there are some people who drink enormous quantities and claim they can't feel a thing.

This is the same phenomenon that physicians observe when they prescribe sleeping pills for a patient. It is extremely hard to measure individual sensitivity beforehand. For example, one person will take half a sleeping pill, sleep for two days, and be groggy on the third. Most people will take a sleeping pill and it will work to a greater or lesser degree. And some people say sleeping pills have no effect—or even opposite effects—unless they take three or four.

Clearly, there are people who are very sensitive to particular chemicals, while others are less so. When looking

at a particular food or spice, remember that its effects may
be different for different people even though they are given
the identical amount.

The second consideration concerns the basic nature of
food and drugs, and harks back to the insight that the
difference between a therapeutic and a toxic effect may be
just a matter of dosage. For example, alcohol is considered
to be a physiological depressant and everybody has seen a
person who is drunk lying immobile, yet there is a dosage
range at which it makes people high—lively, talkative, and
excited.

Similarly, a small amount of foods that are depressants
may produce opposite effects. The explanation probably lies
in the fact that the latest evolutionary addition to our brains
is inhibition. The last added is likely to be the first affected,
so any depressant tends to reduce inhibition first, allowing
excitation to come through.

Most people find that MSG (monosodium glutamate)
tends to make them feel sleepy or sluggish. However, some
people report that it tends to make them jittery or overactive
at first. The effects described on the following charts must
be considered only as tendencies, since people react in such
different ways. Why this is so is not known. Certainly basic
constitution and nervous system type has much to do with
it. But there is more, since people may differ in their
responses from week to week, even from day to day. The
following charts should be viewed with this in mind.

COMMON SPICES	MAJOR CHEMICAL (IF KNOWN)	DOMINANT EFFECTS
Allspice (Pimiento, Jamaica Pepper)	eugenol	mild relaxant
Cardamom	eucalyptol, sabinene	relaxant

COMMON SPICES	MAJOR CHEMICAL (IF KNOWN)	DOMINANT EFFECTS
Cayenne Pepper (in Tabasco sauce)	capsaicin, capsico	mild stimulant
Chili Powder		mild stimulant
Cinnamon	cinnamaldehyde	mild stimulant
Cloves	eugenol	mild relaxant
Ginger	gingerol	mild stimulant
Mace	myristin	stimulant
Monosodium Glutamate	MSG	causes drowsiness, headache; associated with depression
Nutmeg	myristin	stimulant in low doses; high doses cause hallucinations
Pepper	piperine, myristin	mild stimulant
Saffron	picrocrocin	mild stimulant
Tumeric (in curry)	at least ten compounds— major: curcumin, turmerone	mild stimulant
Vanilla	pinene	mild stimulant

COMMON HERBS	MAJOR CHEMICAL (IF KNOWN)	DOMINANT EFFECTS
Anise	anethole, methylchavicol	relaxant
Basil	eucalyptol, methylchavicol	mild relaxant
Borage		stimulant; associated with antidepressant effects

COMMON HERBS	MAJOR CHEMICAL (IF KNOWN)	DOMINANT EFFECTS
Caraway	carvone, carvol, limonene	mild stimulant
Celery Seed	limonene, sedanolide	relaxant; used in cases of menstrual cramps
Coriander	coriandrol, pinene	mild stimulant
Dill		mild sedative
Fennel	fenchone, pinene	mild stimulant
Garlic	alliin, allicin	mild stimulant; antibiotic actions
Hops	lupulone, humulone	sedative
Horseradish	sinigrin	mild stimulant in low doses
Juniper Berries	juniperine, pinene	diuretic, mild stimulant
Marjoram	terpinene	mild sedative actions reported
Parsley	apiol	slight sedative; aspirinlike effects
Poppy Seeds	opiumlike	mild sedative
Rosemary	borneol, eucalyptol, pinene	stimulant known to be associated with aiding memory
Spearmint, Peppermint	menthol, curvone	mild stimulant
Thyme	thymol, pinene	mild stimulant
Wormwood	thujyl, thujone	relaxant, sedative

COMMON VEGETABLES	MAJOR CHEMICAL	DOMINANT EFFECTS
Beans—Broad Bean Pods	tyramine	stimulant

COMMON VEGETABLES	MAJOR CHEMICAL	DOMINANT EFFECTS
Beans—Soybeans	thiouracil-like	depresses thyroid in large, continuous doses; depressant
Cabbage	antithyroid	depressant if taken in excess over period of time
Carrots	estrogenlike	very mild sexual stimulant for women, calming for men
Celery	diuretic chemicals	mildly calming
Lettuce	lactucin	mild sedative
Peas	antithyroid	depressant if taken in excess or continuously
Potatoes	low level of scopolamine alkaloids	sleep-inducing
Seaweed	high in iodine	thyroid stimulant particularly if thyroid is less active due to iodine deficiency
Sprouts	hordenine	mild stimulant
Yams	steroid sapogenin	estrogenlike actions

COMMON FRUITS AND NUTS	MAJOR CHEMICAL	DOMINANT EFFECTS
Anise Fruit	anethole, methylchavicol	relaxant; some estrogenlike effects

COMMON FRUITS AND NUTS	MAJOR CHEMICAL	DOMINANT EFFECTS
Areca Nut (Betel Nut)	arecoline alkaloids	stimulant
Banana	fats, tryptophan	sleep-inducing
Kola Nut	caffeinelike	stimulant
Mango	anacardic acid	tranquility; associated with mild antidepressant action (beware of overdose or allergy)
Palm Kernel	palmitin	estrogenlike actions
Persimmon	caffeinelike	stimulant
Pineapple	tryptophan	relaxant
Pomegranate	pelleterine alkaloids	seeds have some estrogenlike actions; associated with spiritual states
Watermelon	cucurbocitrin	calming, blood pressure lowering, diuretic

COMMON ANIMAL PRODUCTS

FOOD	MAJOR CHEMICAL (IF KNOWN)	DOMINANT EFFECTS
Cheese (aged)	tyramine	stimulant
Cheese (processed)	tryptophan, lecithin	sleep-inducing; mild sedative

COMMON ANIMAL PRODUCTS

FOOD	MAJOR CHEMICAL (IF KNOWN)	DOMINANT EFFECTS
Chicken	some tryptophan	mild stimulant; can have adrenaline-like and steroid actions depending on breeding and slaughter technique
Chicken Livers	tyramine	can be stimulatory
Eggs	high choline, lecithin	mildly sleep-inducing
Fish	high in iodine	maintains thyroid; stimulant
Fugu (Japanese Puffer Fish)	glandular-stimulating	aphrodisiac qualities
Lobster	steroids, GABA (gamma hydroxybutyric acid)	tend toward drowsiness
Meat (Beef)	high in tryptophan and many other amino acids	usually induces sleep and lethargy unless taken in small quantities
Milk	high in tryptophan	tend toward sleep-inducing, relaxing, drowsiness
Oysters and Other Shellfish	steroids, iodine, zinc	tend toward thyroid stimulation, sexual stimulation
Pickled Herring	tyramine	stimulant
Turkey	highest in tryptophan	drowsiness, sleep-inducing

COMMON BEVERAGES (NON-ALCOHOLIC)	MAJOR CHEMICAL (IF KNOWN)	DOMINANT EFFECTS
Camomile Tea		relaxant
Catnip Tea	nepatalic acid and related compounds	relaxant
Chocolate Drinks	theobromine	mild stimulant; possible sexuality enhancement
Coca-Cola	caffeine, other alkaloids from coca leaf, kola nut	stimulant; slightly euphoric relaxant
Coffee	caffeine	stimulant
Ephedra Tea (Mormon Tea)	ephedrine	mild stimulant; airway opener; sexual stimulant in men
Ginger Ale (with Ginger)	gingerol	mild stimulant
Ginseng Tea	steroids	probable enhanced stress resistance; mild sexual stimulant
Khat Tea (Yemenite Tea)	ephedrine, amphetaminelike	stimulant
maté	caffeine	stimulant
Peppermint and Spearmint Teas	menthol, thymol	mild stimulant
Sage Tea		mild sedative
Salep	caffeinelike substances	stimulant
Sarsaparilla	steroid compounds	possible mild sexual stimulant in men
Valerian Tea	valerine, chatinine alkaloids	sedative, relaxant, sleep inducer

TYRAMINE-CONTAINING FOODS: Stimulants and Talk Inducers (beware of headaches!)

Aged Cheese

Pickled Herring

Chicken Livers

Chianti Wine

Sour Cream

Beer

Very Ripe Bananas, Avocados

Chocolate

Soy Sauce

Yeast Extracts

Yogurt

Sherry

Canned Figs

Some Champagne

Aged beef

FOODS CONTAINING CAFFEINE AND SIMILAR ALKALOIDS: Stimulants and Talk Inducers

Coffee

Ephedra Tea

Coca Leaf and Coca-Cola

Khat Tea

Chocolate

Tea

Kola Nuts

Chicle as in chewing gum

Peppermint

VITAMINS AND FOODS
(Many foods not listed have lesser amounts.)

FOODS HIGH IN VITAMIN A

Carrots

Apricots

Yellow Melons

Peaches

Prunes

Butter

Egg Yolks

Liver

Liver Oil

Parsley

Spinach

Dandelion Greens

Mint

Butter

FOODS HIGH IN VITAMIN E

Oils (Cottonseed, Soybean,
  Safflower, Wheat Germ,
  Coconut, Olive, Peanut)
Sunflower Seeds
Barley

Soybeans
Peanuts
Yeast

FOODS HIGH IN VITAMIN B$_1$ (Thiamine)

Wheat Germ
Rice Bran
Soybean Flour
Yeast
Ham

Most Nuts (Almonds, Brazil,
  Cashews, Pecans, Walnuts,
  Chestnuts, Peanuts)
Barley
Rice
Oats
Potatoes

FOODS HIGH IN VITAMIN B$_6$

Liver
Herring
Salmon
Walnuts

Peanuts
Wheat Germ
Brown Rice
Yeast

FOODS HIGH IN VITAMIN B$_{12}$

Kidneys
Liver
Brains
Hearts

Egg Yolks
Clams, Sardines, Salmon,
  Crabs, Oysters, Herring

FOODS HIGH IN VITAMIN C

Lemons
Oranges
Strawberries
Guava
Kiwi Fruit
Chili (green)
Papayas
Broccoli

Brussels Sprouts
Horseradish
Kale
Parsley
Rose Hips
Spinach
Beet Greens

FOODS HIGH IN VITAMIN B$_3$ (Niacin)

Peanuts
Rice Bran
Liver
Hearts

Rabbit, Turkey, Chicken
Tuna, Halibut, Swordfish
Yeast

FOODS HIGH IN ZINC

Oysters
Herring
Clams

Liver
Wheat Bran
Wheat Germ

FOODS HIGH IN MAGNESIUM

Milk
Wheat and whole grains

Most Nuts (Peanuts, Cashews,
Walnuts, Almonds)

FOODS HIGH IN CALCIUM

Milk and Dairy Products
Egg Shells

Bone Meal
Hearts

HIGH-POWERED VEGETABLES
OLD-WORLD HALLUCINOGENIC PLANTS
(FROM EUROPE, ASIA, AUSTRALIA, AFRICA)

Fly Agaric Mushroom
Agara
Kwashi
Galangal
Marijuana
Turkestan Mint
Syrian Rue

Kanna
Belladonna
Henbane
Mandrake
Dhatura (Datura, night-shade)
Iboga

NEW-WORLD HALLUCINOGENIC PLANTS
(FROM NORTH, CENTRAL,
AND SOUTH AMERICA; WEST INDIES)

Puffball Fungus
Psilocybin Mushroom
Stropharia Mushroom
Sweet Flag
Virolas
Jurema
Yopo
Vilca
Genista
Mescal Bean
Colorines (Erythrina species)
Piule
Ayahuasca, Caapi, Yage
Shanshi
Sinicuichi

San Pedro Cactus
Peyote Cactus
Morning Glory (Ololiuqui)
Hierba Loca, Taglli (species of
   Pernettya)
Hojas de la Pastora (*Salvia
   divinorum*)
Borrachera
Arbol de los Brujos
   (sorcerers' tree)
Chiric Sanango (*Brunfelsia*)
Datura (Nightshade),
   including Jimson Weed
Culebra Borrachero
   (Methysticodendron
   amnesium)
Shanin (*Petunia violacea*)
Keule Fruit and Nutmeg
Taique
Tupa (*Lobelia*)
Zacatechichi

5 ⌒ Foods for Religion

Food and religion have been closely linked throughout recorded history. Depending upon how important the production of a mystical consciousness is to a society, some foods have been either revered or banned. Our own society has leaned over backwards to outlaw those foods, mostly vegetables, that alter consciousness. A good example is the coca plant, a vitamin-rich vegetable with strength-giving and mood-elevating properties.

There has been a great recurrence of interest in the coca plant. One Harvard researcher, Dr. Andrew Weil, points out that it has been an important dietary adjunct of Indians in nutritionally deficient areas. It has been an honored part of the South American diet for centuries.

The history of the coca plant, source of cocaine and many other alkaloids, is deeply intertwined with the Inca religions. Coca was seen as a gift of the Earth Mother to man meant to increase his endurance and ability to withstand hardship. In fact, the coca plant is part of the symbol of Peru. But it has been banned in many parts of the world. Coca is not alone in that regard; coffee, tea, chocolate, alcohol, tomatoes, and even the humble potato have experienced the same onslaught.

The Incas called the coca plant "a living manifestation of divinity and the places of its growth a sanctuary where all mortals should bend the knee," and said, "Our God first this coca sent/Endowed with leaves of wond'rous nourishment."

Legends abound about this vegetable and its power. The history of coca sheds light on the nature of the divine in one culture and of the secular in another. It is remarkable that a plant held sacred in one culture is banned in another. The same situation prevails with regard to the mescal cactus, revered by the Aztecs and Mexican Indians, as well as the psilocybin mushroom. In fact, the mushroom is named Teonactl which means literally, "flesh of the gods."

Tea-for-Tao

Tea has figured prominently in many Oriental religious rites. The exact origin of tea is uncertain, but it seems to have been in China. As with coffee, there are many stories that explain the discovery of the virtues of this liquid, which comes from steeping the leaves of the tea plant (*Camellia sinensis*) in water. One well-known myth has it that Daruma, the Buddhist saint, wished to meditate for ten years and during that time, he said, he would not fall asleep. However, he did indeed fall asleep after two years and, upon awakening, his shame was so great that he tore off his eyelids since they had closed. Where the eyelids fell the tea plant arose, and it was imbued with the property of inducing wakefulness.

The earliest detailed book about tea dates from the seventh century A.D. and, true to the deliberate and reverent spirit of the Taoists, each step in the preparation was described in an orderly and ritualistic way. This work, by the poet Lu Yu (the patron saint of tea), was called *Ch'a Ching* ("The Classic of Tea"), and delves into exquisite detail regarding the cultivation and harvesting as well as the serving of tea. Lu Yu believed in the need for great care in dealing with tea, and insisted that all gatherers bathe before picking tea and not eat pungent food to avoid imparting unpleasant odors to the leaves.

One little-known but important fact included in his work is that at that time, the Chinese customarily added salt to tea. Because of the diuretic properties of tea (water and salt losses via the kidney), the taking of salt can be seen as supplementing this loss. Perhaps the tea at Chinese restaurants plays an important role in ridding the body of the large quantities of salt (and monosodium glutamate) in Chinese food.

The pleasant effects of tea actually led to the cult of Teaism which was founded to emphasize the beautiful among the sordid facts of everyday existence. Cultists worshiped the "Queen of the Camellias" and reveled in the warm stream of amber liquid filled with feeling and sympathy which the plant gave to man.

Naturally, as tea spread throughout the world there was opposition to it. In London, it was denounced as a filthy custom by Henry Sayville in 1678. Jonas Hanway, in an essay on tea written almost seventy-five years later, said that men seemed to lose their stature and women their beauty through the use of tea.

Tea did remain in Britain despite the few naysayers and teetotalers, and became increasingly important. In fact, the English never became coffee drinkers to the same extent that they took tea.

What are some of the effects of tea? Samuel Johnson found it a fascinating plant food and said, "With tea I amused the evening, with tea solaced the midnight and with tea welcomed the morning." He is said to have consumed at least twenty cups of tea daily.

The active components of tea include the alkaloid theophylline, which is a relative of caffeine, but which also opens the airways in the lungs and hastens the passage of urine. Do not conclude, however, that the only active ingredient in tea is theophylline, which varies in amount from type to type. Tea has a high tannin content and contains some trace oils as well as other alkaloids that can account for the differing sensations tea drinkers experience from varieties of tea. Also, the true tea drinker is stimulated by the smell as well as the color.

Tea stimulates the central nervous system and thus is an awakener. To a lesser extent than coffee, tea induces talk. To a much greater extent, however, tea induces a relaxed—even euphoric—state.

In the words of the poet Lu T'ung:

> The first cup moistens my lips and throat, the second
> cup breaks my loneliness, the third cup searches my
> barren entrails, but to find therein some five thousand
> volumes of odd ideographs, the fourth cup raises a
> slight perspiration, all the wrong of life passes through
> my pores. At the fifth cup, I am purified. The sixth
> cup calls me to the realms of the immortals, the
> seventh cup—Ah, but I could take no more. I only
> feel the breath of cool wind that rises in my sleeves.
> Let me ride on this sweet breeze and waft away thither.

Perhaps the American habit of a quick cup of coffee or tea actually deprives people of the real effects of tea in terms of enhancing their mood and increasing appreciation of beauty.

The ultimate in appreciation of tea is probably seen in the elaborate ceremony in Japan where the monks drink tea out of a communal bowl with the formality of a holy sacrament. The profound influence that tea exerts upon the personality can be seen in a Japanese expression. While we say of a dull or lackluster person, "He lacks vim or vigor," they say, "He has no tea in him."

Tea Types

There are three types of traditional tea: black, oolong, and green. The differences reside in the manner by which the tea leaf is processed. In green tea, the leaf is boiled soon after picking, which stops certain enzyme processes of the leaf. Black tea owes its color to a longer period of time in which enzymes act. The oolong teas have an intermediate amount of enzyme activity, so that the dark color of the black tea leaf is not reached. Oxidation is the process that turns the leaf black, but it is often erroneously referred to as fermentation. Tea grading is thought to relate to the quality of tea, but in fact this process really only separates tea according to leaf size. For example, the term "orange pekoe" only describes the size and shape of the leaves.

Tea tasters list at least thirty descriptive words regarding tea. The tea in tea bags tends to be inferior in almost all these measures. The principal reason for this is that the apportioning of tea in a small bag leads to its more rapidly going stale. People who use only tea bags may never have had a true tea experience.

Holy Herbs and Spices

Much prized by the Romans and termed either "devil's dung" or "food of the gods" is the asafetida, from the roots of the *Ferula asafoetida*. There are many compounds in it, including pinene and vanillin, both stimulants. In large doses, the pinene induces delirium and hallucinations. It bears mentioning that the fermented asafetida is much stronger and was once said to be worth its weight in silver.

This is probably the "dove's dung" referred to in the Bible (II Kings 6:26) where the inflationary trend of this prized food is decried. Dr. Alfred Stillé, Professor of Medicine at the University of Pennsylvania Medical School in 1874, recommended it highly to "provide vigor without nervous excitement." It is still used in Asia as a condiment, although its odor is strong and repugnant to some people.

In Biblical times, holy oils usually included a base of olive oil with myrrh, frankincense, sweet calamus, and cassia (cinnamon) added. When used in anointing, the precious olive oil and the sweet-smelling liquid contributed to the religious effect. However, the myrrh, one of the gifts brought to the Christ Child, seems to have some mild stimulant effects. The sweet calamus contains some steroidlike substances. Of course, the olive oil is a good source of the essential fatty acids.

Anise, also mentioned frequently in the Bible, is the dried fruit of the *Pimpinella anisum* and has mild stimulant effects as well as some estrogen effects. The distillation of the fermented fruit and juice leads to a prized liquor.

Spikenard is another valuable herb written of in the Bible. It probably refers to the herb valerian, which has sedating qualities and was used in World War I to treat shell shock.

The frankincense (or olibanum) brought to the Christ Child is the gum resin from the *Boswellia carteri* (or birdwood). Like the asafetida, it contains pinene, a mild stimulant, as well as a whole range of polysaccharides (sugars and starches linked together). The polysaccharides may exert an effect as yet undetermined.

Sacred Plants

The druids were a tightly knit order with secret codes. They were the priests and soothsayers of the Celts prior to the introduction of Christianity to Britain. Their sacred remedy involved the spores of the club-moss. This fine yellow powder contains a substance called selagnine, which can have hallucinogenic effects. The druids felt this remedy enhanced psychic powers.

Yage, ololiuqui, and other mind-altering plants figure prominently in South American religious rites. One little-known plant—the manace— deserves more study. From the dried root of the Brazilian shrub *Brunfelsia hopeana,* it reportedly has been used for many years for its aphrodisiac qualities and as an aid in shamanism. The plant contains many alkaloidlike substances, and from their chemical structures, some psychedelic effects could be predicted.

As Dr. Albert Hoffman said about religion and the use of psychedelic substances, "another reason for the incidence of religious experiences is the fact that the very core of the human mind is connected with God. This deepest root of our consciousness which in the normal state is hidden by superficial rational activities of the mind may become revealed by the action of the psychedelic drug."

Like many others, Dr. Hoffman feels that psychedelic agents may be enlightening in the sense that under the influence of these drugs "we become conscious of the entire complex of interhuman and intercosmic relations with an immediacy, an intimacy and a realism that might otherwise happen only in spontaneous ecstatic states and to a very few blessed people." (From an interview with Dr. Hoffman printed in *High Times,* March 1976.)

The similarity between Dr. Hoffman's comments and the description of "seeing" that Don Juan, the Yaqui Indian, taught Carlos Castañeda might be related to the mushrooms and cactus eaten. Like Dr. Hoffman, Carl Jung felt that man has a religious center within him. He postulated that if all religions were suddenly abolished along with current memory of them, within a century they would all arise again, although in different forms depending on the culture. Plants and plant products that stimulate this religious center have been prized because of their assistance in worship. Food and drink are a part of many religious rites. Before laughing at a Mexican Indian who feels that the god Mescalito is in the cactus, we must remember the Christian sacraments. Christians symbolically eat and drink of Christ.

The religious consciousness tends to be antithetical to our society. It postulates forces we cannot see, beliefs that go against the rationalist grain. Even further, it provides a threat to a scientific society since this consciousness is often at variance with the existing framework.

The existing framework is a local affair. Where it allows concepts of magic and voodoo, there seems to be enough evidence of magic and voodoo that people maintain their beliefs and fears. There are isolated pockets of such practices in the United States. For example, black people outside of New Orleans believe in a form of voodoo and see evidence of spells working. Our framework cannot explain any of these phenomena except by using a blanket term such as hysteria or suggestion.

Religion is closely tied to mysticism. While we have not developed a real mystical tradition or movement in our country, there are some signs that religion and mysticism will coalesce. New religious groups with their devoted members offer evidence of this, and a variety of "new age" consciousness movements have a mystical base. Descriptions of mystical experiences have been recorded for centuries. The experience of cosmic consciousness has not been explained but seems to be associated with the religious conversion experience. Though we can't say for sure what this experience is, it can be mimicked with some hallucinogenic vegetables such as the mescal cactus and the psilocybin mushroom.

Fasting: The "Internal" Diet

Total fasting may induce highly introspective states, and spare diets have been a part of religious orders and characteristic of many religious leaders. As Matthew (4:1) writes,

"Then Jesus was led up by the spirit into the wilderness to be tempted by the devil. And ... he fasted forty days and forty nights ..." John the Baptist's diet was described in Matthew 3:4: "... and his food was locusts and wild honey."

The fast has been associated with introspection and religious illumination from Jesus to St. Augustine, who wrote of his fasts, to modern-day religious leaders.

There has been increasing interest in the mental changes brought about by fasting, particularly when recent reports have demonstrated that a reduction in symptoms of depression can result from a simple fast of two or three days. The decrease in the sympathetic nervous system (which is high in stress and anxiety) might account for some of these observations. Also, in sensitive people, choline can exacerbate depressions (as reported in *Lancet* in 1976 by Dr. C. Tamminga and his colleagues). Thus, for these people choline reduction (as through fasting) might be helpful and might help explain the reduction in symptoms of depression. There are some fascinating reasons for why this may be so, and analysis of what occurs in the body during fasting may offer insights into how fasting can aid in healing activities.

Foodstuffs of the Brain

Normally when glucose (simple sugar) is available the brain will use it for energy almost exclusively. But when the intake of food is stopped, glucose stores rapidly become depleted. Some glucose is available through the breakdown of body tissues and proteins, but the amount is not sufficient to keep the brain functioning at a high degree of alertness. So what happens? The brain begins to use the breakdown products of fats, called ketones, for its energy. After prolonged fasting (more than twenty to thirty days), an equilibrium is established where approximately 75 percent of the energy comes from ketones and 25 percent comes from available glucose. In terms of fuel for the brain, it appears that there is a minimal level of energy—approximately 25 percent—that must come from glucose. Literally speaking, the "fats burn in the fire of glucose."

In fasting there is total body compensation to conserve. For example, thyroid function diminishes, reducing the basal metabolic rate (the minimum number of calories necessary for body functioning). This also comes about because thyroid hormone is made from the amino acid tyrosine—as supplies of tyrosine are reduced, hormone production is reduced. Also, the activity of the sympathetic nervous system, which controls "fight and flight," is reduced. Thus there is less motivation for fighting and less energy for flight—generally a more peaceful state occurs.

Meanwhile, back in the brain, let's look at the other systems. It has been well demonstrated that the two major parts of the involuntary nervous system tend to balance each other. The sympathetic nervous system (fight and flight) is balanced by the parasympathetic nervous system (the housekeeping system having to do with secretion, glandular activity, blood flow, etc.). States of parasympathetic (or cholinergic) excess have been correlated with depressive states, whereas sympathetic nervous system excesses are correlated with states of anxiety. As the sympathetic nervous system decreases in fasting, anxiety also decreases, resulting in calmness, increased introspection, and the kind of internal quiet necessary for religious experiences. The parasympathetic nervous system is also decreased in fasting. The parasympathetic system depends to a great extent upon the introduction of choline and lecithin into the body. When these supplies are shut off, the parasympathetic nervous system slows down. When ketones are used for the brain's energy, the rate of acetylcholine production is much slower than when glucose is used as the fuel.

Thus, while both systems are reduced, the parasympathetic seems to be reduced more, leading to sympathetic nervous system predominance. Once the level of the anxiety component of the sympathetic nervous system is reduced, we are left with a balance of the other effects—namely, a feeling of well-being. This feeling of well-being has been termed the "fasting high."

There is also another reason for the fasting high which is slightly different from the mechanism described above and probably acts conjointly. The late Dr. Harold Himwich, a legendary figure in brain research, discovered that as patients are given insulin shock treatments for mental illness, the brain goes through various phases. In insulin shock therapy, a dose of insulin is given to a patient, the blood sugar level falls rapidly, and a comalike state occurs. Then, after a short period of time, glucose is given to the patient and he or she wakes up. The interesting finding is that after awakening many of the symptoms of schizophrenia as well as serious depression are alleviated.

As Dr. Himwich plotted out the various changes that occurred with insulin shock he became aware that the sympathetic-parasympathetic balance was changing. He noted that without any particular state of stress there is a parasympathetic predominance—a settled, undisturbed patient with a slow heart rate, watery salivation, comfortable position. If the patient is disturbed quickly, there is a sudden sympathetic nervous system surge which overcomes the parasympathetic dominance.

The parasympathetic dominance occurs in the state of full awareness and full function of the brain. The most advanced portion of our human brain is the cortical layer and the most advanced portion of that is an inhibitory component. It is this inhibitory component that has to do with control, an advanced function. However, when the inhibitory com-

ponent becomes too powerful there are depressive reactions—excess inhibitions. Apparently, man has always
searched for ways to at least temporarily disconnect the
inhibitory component because this state of release is
pleasurable. For example, he has tried to depress the inhibition with alcohol or other drugs, or to override the
inhibition with stimulatory drugs or worldly stimulation.

If the brain is impaired, loss of function occurs in
descending order. That is, the most advanced function is
diminished first. As the brain switches over to fatty acid
metabolism there is some decrease in efficiency. The inhibitory component's function is diminished first. It is still there,
but is not as powerful. And the inhibitory functioning, which
is associated with the parasympathetic nervous system, is
diminished along with the functioning of the parasympathetic
nervous system. The result is a slight euphoria—the euphoria
of release—much like the high that occurs as the first stage
of alcohol intoxication. Perhaps we are too frequently in the
grip of overinhibitory systems.

Relation Between Fasting and Healing

Many diseases seem to be associated with states of excess
parasympathetic nervous system stimulation (excess cholinergic stimulation). For example, ulcer disease, with its excess
acid production, is treated by cutting the parasympathetic
nerves to the stomach. Depression seems to be associated
with an excessive parasympathetic nervous system reaction.
Just think of a grief reaction—pupils constricted, watery eyes,
coughing, excess mucus; sluggishness; susceptibility to in-
fection, particularly pulmonary. Energy level is impaired, the
joy is out of life. Everything is "black"—a useful expression
since the eyes are so constricted that very little light is let in;
compare it with "wide-eyed with excitement," or "you light
up my life," or "I feel so much brighter."

In a state where the functioning of the parasympathetic nervous system is diminished, there is a corresponding diminution in the symptoms of diseases that appear to reflect parasympathetic nervous system dominance—for example, depression, grief, ulcer disease.

At the same time there are particular disorders that reflect predominance of the sympathetic nervous system— hypertension, backaches, nervous tension, etc. In fasting the functioning of the sympathetic nervous system is also reduced, though it is dominant over the parasympathetic. This state is associated with a reduction of symptoms that seem to represent sympathetic nervous system excesses. Thus blood pressure is lower, anxiety may increase, muscular tension is less.

Fasting and the Religious Experience

As a result of the complex changes described above, the individual is able to attain a clarity of mind in which, for whatever biochemical reason, he is open to profound religious experiences.

Is the mystical and religious experience always around us but rarely appreciated because we don't have the proper internal quiet? Or is it more of a biochemical happening reflecting a simple metabolic difference? This question is moot. Having had a religious experience myself I can attest to its reality.

What are such experiences? There are constant elements in reported religious experiences. These seem to be a feeling of rebirth, a feeling of illumination and moral exaltation, a feeling of being chosen, and a sense of immortality and the continuity of life.

Many who have experienced this state seem to have gone into a retreat involving isolation, fasting, and meditation. Sometimes a brief blindness follows an intense subjective experience of light. Often there are bright clouds described and an overpowering feeling of love and the presence of God. Speech may be impaired during the event. While the extreme cosmic consciousness has apparently been experienced by very few, many people sense some of this feeling during prayer.

Mystics have considered the source of this feeling to be the so-called third eye, the pineal gland. While Descartes believed the pineal gland to be the seat of the soul, for many years it was looked upon in men as having very little function. Some animals such as frogs and lizards actually have a prominent third eye on their foreheads, but in man, this structure has receded within the brain.

In an old Egyptian myth, the god of health, Horus, lost an eye and it was replaced by Thoth, the god of wisdom, who located the eye within. From that point, this third eye has been associated with wisdom and to some extent with the process of "seeing" in the broadest sense (perhaps the kind of seeing that Don Juan spoke of to Carlos Castañeda).

This third eye symbol of wisdom has been represented on the back of the U.S. dollar bill—on the left is a pyramid with a single eye.

The pineal organ is rich in a compound called serotonin, a "chemical messenger" which allows transmission from one area of the brain to another, and which has been linked with states of altered consciousness. There is mounting evidence that the pineal gland, which twenty years ago was thought to be without function, is associated with a religious consciousness.

The pineal gland also seems to be closely associated with adjustments to light and darkness and in this way seems to be an organ of our adaptation. In addition, it relates to puberty in still unexplained ways. The earlier puberty experienced by girls in tropical regions where the sun shines longer is believed to be linked with the pineal.

Certain foods rich in the precursor amino acid of

serotonin, tryptophan, seem to be associated with altered states of consciousness and perhaps a religious sense. Buddha was sitting under a fig tree when he received the enlightenment; the fig is a good source of tryptophan. Perhaps he had eaten quite a quantity before resting. The fig has been called "the guide of men to civilization." Other foods rich in serotonin or tryptophan include peanuts, pineapples, bananas, and dates. The Saracens called the date the "King of Fruits."

The tryptophan and serotonin metabolisms seem closely associated with sexual functions and feelings of love—both spiritual and physical. The removal of the pineal delays puberty. Tumors of the pineal gland causing overactivity result in precocious puberty and hypersexuality. The sexual function should not be considered purely "animal" in nature. In fact, in the holy and mystical kabbala, the book of the Jewish mystical tradition, the sexual activity is seen as a holy act—melding the two spirits together—and those who do not procreate are denied access to Paradise.

That the sexual and love functions are close is not surprising. Both might relate to the pineal gland, and religious exaltation is often an experience of love apart from sexual love. The chemical sequence is: the amino acid tryptophan is converted into serotonin which is then converted into melatonin. Melatonin, one of the hormones of the pineal gland, inhibits sexuality. The more serotonin formed, the greater the likelihood of more melatonin and therefore less sexuality—but perhaps more feelings of love.

The biochemical linkages have not yet been fully explored. However, states of fasting have been shown to result in relative increases in the serotonin and pineal functions. Also certain depressions with anxiety have been linked to low serotonin levels in the brain. What does this mean in a practical dietary sense? For a heightened religious experience fasting is an aid. But fasting is not necessary if the following diet is observed.

A Diet for Religion

Is fasting the only way to reach a state of inner calm, reduced anxiety, greater introspection? The answer is no! But as discussed in chapter 3, diets have to be tailored for desired states. The diet for introspection and religious experience is far from the diet needed by, for example, a competitive athlete.

Basic Principles of the Religious Diet

To reach a state of religious consciousness we must through the use of food create a sympathetic nervous system dominance over the parasympathetic nervous system without creating excesses in the sympathetic nervous system. Basically, this is also the "diet of healing." Because it is a diet for a particular purpose, it should not be considered a continuous diet—over a long period of time, it would bring about nutritional deficiencies. However, it is a safe diet for a period of three weeks for a well-nourished person.

PRINCIPLE #1: Use Foods to Suppress the Parasympathetic Nervous System.
A. *Decrease choline intake.* Choline has been shown to influence the formation of acetylcholine, the nerve transmitter of the parasympathetic nervous system. Large amounts of choline are present in the following foods:

> egg yolks (2 grams per 100 grams)
> meats (600 mg per 100 grams)
> fish (200 mg per 100 grams)
> cereals (100 mg per 100 grams)

These foods should be entirely avoided to substantially reduce choline.
Foods to use: fruits
　　　　　leafy vegetables

Vegetables to avoid: legumes (e.g., peas, beans)

B. *Decrease lecithin intake.* Lecithin is a type of fat used extensively as a food additive because it helps to emulsify foods. Check labels. Lecithin is directly associated with the formation of acetylcholine. Avoid animal fats and milk products.

PRINCIPLE #2: Avoid Foods That Stimulate the Sympathetic Nervous System.
Do not use coffee, tea, or cola beverages. Do not use refined sugar. Do not eat meat or meat products.

PRINCIPLE #3: Increase Tryptophan Foods Such as Nuts and Pineapple. Avoid bananas, fermented food, and avocados. Avoid dairy products, which have a good deal of tryptophan but also a lot of choline.
In summary, foods for the religious diet are:

1. Fruits
2. Leafy vegetables
3. Nuts

All others should either be avoided or substantially reduced. The astute observer might point out that after a careful biochemical approach we have arrived at just the diet that Buddha recommended for purification.

6 Foods for Sleep or Wakefulness

Sleep is a basic need for man as fundamental as eating, but variations in amount of sleep a person needs may be great. To understand more about it, we must concern ourselves with ordinary sleep, dreaming sleep, and productive sleep.

Let us start with a normal person—call her Mary Smith—and follow her as she first feels tired, then gets ready for bed, and after about fifteen minutes "falls asleep." Gradually her electroencephalogram (a reading of electrical brain waves) goes from a random low-voltage pattern to a more regular pattern of fairly rapid waves. After about ten minutes the brain waves become slower and more pronounced, proceeding to what is termed stage 4 sleep where the brain waves are almost entirely long, slow delta waves. This sort of sleep seems to be needed for body repair processes.

After about seventy minutes, an interesting phenomenon occurs. The brain waves start getting faster and seem to be approaching the pattern that occurred immediately after Mary fell asleep. At this time, rapid eye movements (REMS) begin, indicating the start of the first dream. During this first REM period, which may last only five or ten minutes, there seems to be an overall body activation. The pulse rate increases, the blood pressure fluctuates, the respiratory rate becomes more irregular, the glands become more active and, in men, an erection may occur.

After five or ten minutes of dreams, Mary will repeat the cycle, reaching stage 4 sleep, and in another seventy or eighty minutes will return to a REM state. This pattern goes on through the night, but the REM periods get progressively longer. The reason for the REM periods is still a matter of much discussion, but many researchers feel they have something to do with adaptation—sorting and filing new experiences. In new or unusual environments there is initially more REM sleep. On the other hand, the non-REM sleep, particularly the delta-wave sleep, is felt to reflect a need for reparative processes. When people are deprived of sleep for several days, a recording of the recuperative night will show more delta-wave sleep, often with the first one or two REM periods missed entirely. Subsequently, there seems to be a need for catching up on REM sleep.

Productive sleep means getting the most from the least amount of sleep and waking up feeling rested. It also may mean creative, problem-solving sleep. Everybody knows that on one night they may get the same amount of sleep as on another night, but somehow one night has been more "restful" than another. Foods can influence these variations. Foods can mean the difference between getting eight hours of sleep and waking to feel that there has been an eight-hour battle, or getting eight hours or less of refreshing sleep.

What is creative sleep? Everybody has heard the expression "I'll sleep on it," reflecting the problem-solving process that can occur. The great nineteenth-century chemist Kekulé von Stradonitz dreamed about snakes one night, and in the morning, remembering the snakes joining together, he realized he had discovered the structure of the benzene ring. Coleridge reported that the opening lines of "Kubla Khan" came to him in an opium dream.

Because sleep can be of good or poor quality the question "How much sleep does a person need?" becomes meaningless. In fact, there is no evidence that those who sleep for shorter hours have increased illnesses, shorter lives, or any discernible problem except irritability if they get less than their body needs. A man in Australia decided that all he really needed was three hours of sleep nightly, and after ten years, testing revealed him to be a healthy and happy man. History is filled with tales of extremely productive men and women who were able to make use of the time others were sleeping. Napoleon and the great scientist Rudolf Virchow are examples. Thomas Edison deliberately limited his sleep time to four or five hours (sometimes helped by the coca plant). He felt that his light bulb would help people to get less sleep since they could use the night hours more easily.

Most people sleep for about one-third of their lives. Consider: If a person can feel the same sense of well-being, perform well, and sleep two hours less each night, there would be thirty extra days of living each year and more than four extra years between the ages of 20 and 70!

Coffee and Tea

Dr. Israel Bram, a thyroid specialist in Philadelphia, had an interesting hobby related to his curiosity about sleep. During the 1930s he sent questionnaires to people in *Who's Who* dealing with the sleep habits of the famous. Of one hundred fifty-three who responded, seventy reported that coffee before bed made sleep difficult. Those who found that coffee disturbed their sleep included Clarence Darrow, Dorothy Dix, Ernest Hemingway, H. L. Mencken, Margaret Sanger, and Edgar Guest. There is, of course, a psychological aspect—people who say coffee will keep them awake tend to fulfill their prophecy. As Edgar Guest wrote, "I feel that the Human bein' is more potent than the coffee bean." On the other hand, sleep studies show that after caffeine intake there is more of the rapid brain-wave sleep and less of the slow, deep delta-wave sleep which is felt to be a time of body repair. In addition, there is less dream time after caffeine. Paradoxically, excess coffee drinking close to sleep hours may create a need for more sleep.

The same holds true for chocolate and tea, but tea has an additional effect. The theophylline in tea (similar to caffeine, but with some different effects) will produce a slight phase shift. This deserves some explanation. It is accurate to say that "we got rhythm." There are at least one hundred body functions that undergo daily predictable fluctuations. For example, the temperature of a person seems to fall when bedtime is nearing and reaches a low point at about 3 or 4 A.M. Then, almost as if the body is preparing for the day, the temperature begins to rise.

In those who habitually awaken at 8 A.M. the temperature is on the upswing then and reaches a high point about 9 or 10 A.M. Taking tea seems to shift the pattern. For example, two or three cups of tea before bed will result in a slightly later temperature rise so that if we awaken at the usual time our bodies would have a feeling of inadequate sleep and would require a longer time to feel ready for the day. Such phase retardation, as it has been called, has more than theoretical effects because it bears on performance. When the military ran tests of hand steadiness and reaction time, performance correlated closely with body temperature, being best when the temperature was at its peak. The person who awakens at a low point in his temperature cycle feels fatigued even when sleep has been ample. For example, think of how you might feel if you had to wake up at 4 A.M. if your usual wake-up time is 8 A.M. You would feel chilly and groggy even if you had gone to bed at 8 P.M. and gotten your usual amount of sleep.

Of course we might be able to make use of tea because of just these effects. For example, if we traveled to a location where the time zone was different, we might want to induce this sort of shift. If a person used to awakening in New York at 8 A.M. went to California, he would for at least the first few days tend to wake up at 5 A.M. because that would correspond to his 8 A.M. body time. Tea would tend to change his body rhythm to adjust to California time.

Eating at Bedtime

A bedtime snack is very common and it aids some people in falling asleep. The processes of digestion are related to the parasympathetic nervous system, which is involved in sleep. The snack might contain a sleep-inducing substance like the amino acid tryptophan. However, because of the acid secretion that occurs, people with stomach problems or those who have a hiatus hernia which allows acid to seep upward in the esophagus, resulting in heartburn, may find that a bedtime snack produces needless suffering. Some people have made the correlation of a bedtime snack with nightmares.

James Davis, a U.S. Senator in the 1930s, reported to Dr. Bram that he had great difficulty with sleep after gorging himself at night, most likely due to his stomach disorder. Charles Bartholomew, a notable of the 1900s, also found that food at bedtime caused difficulty in sleeping, and remarked that chocolate in particular kept him awake (that was in the days when chocolate was real).

People without stomach or intestinal disorders generally find a bedtime snack helps induce sleep. This probably relates to the stimulation of the sleep mechanism by food. Urination, a function of that portion of the nervous system, is also relaxing for some. In fact, the writer Gelett Burgess said, "Drinking of considerable water and resultant urination is an excellent producer of sleep. Although one has to awaken more frequently for urination it has a relaxing effect and one falls asleep almost immediately afterwards. In fact, I have often gone to sleep while urinating."

Tryptophan—A Natural Sleep Inducer

Recent investigations have demonstrated that the amino acid tryptophan will induce sleep. This finding is particularly important because the sleep seems to be "natural." Many drugs will produce sleep, but except for one or two exceptions, they all seem to reduce the dream time or otherwise alter the normal sleep pattern. Tryptophan will not do this.

The actions of tryptophan give additional credibility to the old remedy of a glass of warm milk to help insomnia, since milk is a good source of tryptophan. Meats contain tryptophan; a rich source is turkey.

Certain fruits have high levels of tryptophan. For example, the banana is a good source, as is the fig. Perhaps the tryptophan content of the banana has something to do with the slower pace of the tropics. Other foods high in tryptophan (tryptophan is made into serotonin in the body and the serotonin mechanism seems to have much to do with sleep) are pineapples and nuts.

Dr. Michael Jouvet, one of the world's foremost sleep researchers, injected monkeys with a substance that reduced the serotonin content markedly. After thirty hours, the monkeys had complete insomnia which lasted at least another thirty hours. Animals eating a tryptophan-deficient diet develop great irritability and sleep disturbances.

A chemical curiosity is that the proteins called histones, believed to keep the cell-synthesizing processes turned off, are completely lacking in tryptophan. In Edinburgh in 1942, a husband-and-wife investigating team, the Stedmans, found that actively growing tissues seemed to contain fewer histones, although later work showed that they might contain fewer *available* histones. The point is: the tryptophan-containing proteins seemed to be more active in growth processes.

The knowledge of tryptophan as a natural sleep inducer may save many people from sleeping pills. One of the reasons for the poor long-term effects of most sleeping pills is that they artificially suppress activity in the central nervous system. Then, once the pill's effect has worn off, there is often a rebound hyperactivity resulting in a tendency for insomnia the next night. As with a temporary water dam, its removal causes the water to surge with even greater force.

In 1970, Drs. Richard Wyatt, Karl Engelman, and other colleagues reported in the British medical journal *Lancet* that tryptophan was definitely beneficial in stimulating sleep, particularly the slow-wave sleep which seems important for body repair. Since then, numerous studies have confirmed the value of tryptophan. Another important finding is the absence of a drug hangover so common with sleeping pills, particularly the barbiturates. Even when the person doesn't feel the hangover effects, tests of reaction time, vigilance, and complex problem-solving tasks show diminished capability after a barbiturate or barbituratelike pill has been taken the previous night.

Wine and Other Alcohol

Wine has been used from earliest times to induce sleep. In addition to the alcohol content, many of the pigments in red wines seem to produce tranquility.

Hard drinks (those with vodka, gin, Scotch, etc.) exert most of their effects through the alcohol content. On a short-term basis there is probably little harm in inducing sleep this way. But over a longer time period, the rebound hyperexcitability produces more severe insomnia. In this regard, some of the Italian wines, champagnes, and wine punches like sangria act as stimulants and may cause hours of insomnia. This effect can be anticipated in any food that contains protein and then undergoes aging. A wine such as champagne that undergoes a secondary fermentation process can be considered a stimulant. The most relevant chemical reaction seems to be the conversion of tyrosine to tyramine—the same kind of conversion that results in stimulant cheeses.

The effect of hyperexcitability is graphically illustrated by the alcoholic withdrawing from alcohol, hyperexcited and shaking, sometimes in convulsions. F. Scott Fitzgerald described the horrors of insomnia; alcohol was unquestionably a contributor if not the cause. ". . . In a real dark night of the soul it is always three o'clock in the morning day after day." He begged for sleep, "the dear, the cherished one, the lullaby." Yet he previously had found that alcohol would help his sleep disorder. With chemicals that act on the brain there seems to be no "free lunch."

Choline

Because the parasympathetic nervous system, along with serotonin and tryptophan, seems to have an important role in sleep, maintaining the nerve transmitters is important. The major nerve transmitter is acetylcholine, and choline is vital for its formation. Egg yolks are very high in choline, which is also found in meats and, to a lesser extent, in cereals.

It is ironic that Otto Loewi made his Nobel Prize winning discovery of acetylcholine in the following manner: "The night before Easter Sunday of that year [1920] I awoke, turned on the light and jotted down a few notes on a tiny slip of paper. Then I fell asleep again. It occurred to me at six o'clock in the morning that during the night I had written down something very important, but I was unable to decipher the scrawl. The next night at three o'clock the idea returned."

This time he got right up, went to the laboratory and performed a simple experiment. Its results were positive and the foundation for the theory of chemical transmission of the nervous impulse was secure. The fact that he dreamed the same dream at the same time on two successive nights implies that this particular dream element, perhaps a conclusion reached by the brain but unable to break into consciousness, was pressing for release—and quiet sleep allowed this to occur. Perhaps the sleep mechanism, induced by acetylcholine, was related to his finding. That is, he discovered acetylcholine from a dream induced by acetylcholine.

Experiments with acetylcholine stimulation in man have demonstrated that a rapid eye movement dreaming state can be produced almost immediately by an infusion of a substance which raises the acetylcholine. Some recent evidence goes a step further and appears to show that acetylcholine is particularly associated with dreaming sleep, while tryptophan tends to induce more non-dreaming sleep.

Since dietary choline and lecithin will increase levels of acetylcholine, a person with insomnia should ensure that his diet is adequate in substances such as egg yolks, soybean oil, butter, and margarine.

Vitamin C—A Sleepy Vitamin

Vitamin C is involved with the health of the entire body and with multiple organ systems. Severe prolonged deficiency or lack of vitamin C will result in a disease called scurvy. According to some scientists, many of us have a mild deficiency state at all times because we cannot, like some other animals, synthesize vitamin C. Dr. Linus Pauling is probably the strongest advocate of this controversial concept.

While a marked deficiency of vitamin C will produce lassitude and weakness, it also is associated with sleep disturbance. This can be seen most clearly in infants and children who show a great deal of irritability when deficient in vitamin C. Vitamin C also reduces some of the effects of cerebral stimulants such as the amphetamines, demonstrating its role in calming. Dr. Carl Pfeiffer reported in the journal *Psychopharmacology* (1968) that large doses of vitamin C reduce the electrical activity of the brain as measured by an electroencephalogram.

Sources of Vitamin C

HIGH AMOUNTS: citrus fruits, strawberries, cherries, pineapple, tomatoes, chili peppers, collard greens, broccoli.

LOW AMOUNTS: apples, mangoes, cantaloupes.

Almost all fruits and vegetables contain vitamin C, and only a small amount is necessary to prevent scurvy. Still, advocates of vitamin C therapy claim the only way to get adequate amounts is through supplementation by vitamin pills.

Thiamine—See It to Believe It

I first became aware of the potent effects of thiamine (vitamin B_1) in an alcoholic who had been drinking excessively for six years with poor food intake. He arrived at the emergency department in utter confusion with a high level of anxiety. His family said he hadn't slept in days. He was a 35-year-old man, and I had the initial tendency to think that his confusion was due to alcohol withdrawal. However, his absolute memory deficit and inability to recognize me even after a few minutes away from him alerted me to look further. I recalled that a sudden deficiency of thiamine can cause this syndrome, so I administered 100 mg of thiamine into his muscle. In one hour he returned to normal—a dramatic effect I've seen at least five times since in other patients.

An alcoholic who shows such confusion and anxiety should not be dismissed as having "brain rot" or other glib terms indicating alcohol injury of the brain. Thiamine could be his or her answer—at least to reverse some of those acute symptoms, unless they have progressed to irreversibility.

Sources of Thiamine (vitamin B_1)

HIGH AMOUNTS: wheat germ, rice bran, soybean flour, yeast.

MEDIUM AMOUNTS: raisins, beets, potatoes, broccoli, brown rice, most nuts, meats, parsley, peas, eggs, fish.

LOW AMOUNTS: fruits, leafy greens, celery, shrimp, oysters.

Vitamin B_6 (Pyridoxyl Phosphate)— The Major Sleep Vitamin

Probably the most dramatic example of the efficacy of vitamin B_6 is that of a patient being treated for Parkinson's disease who shows signs of excess Dopa (a drug used in treatment) in the nervous system. In such cases, there is marked hypervigilance. Cerebral stimulants such as amphetamines and ritalin also increase the dopamine content of the brain—this is believed to be the major way they promote wakefulness. However, vitamin B_6 will counter the excess effects of dopamine-stimulating substances by aiding in the synthesis of an inhibitory and calming brain chemical, gamma amino butyric acid. Another sign of its calming action is that deficiency of vitamin B_6 is associated with convulsions.

Sources of Vitamin B_6 (Pyridoxyl Phosphate)

HIGH AMOUNTS: liver, herring, salmon, walnuts, peanuts, wheat germ, brown rice, yeast.

MEDIUM AMOUNTS: bananas, avocados, pears, barley, carrots, corn, oats, peas, potatoes, tomatoes, turnips, yams, Brussels sprouts, spinach, soybeans, beef, fish, butter, eggs.

LOW AMOUNTS: citrus fruits, apples, peaches, watermelons, lettuce, onions, cheese, milk, asparagus.

Monosodium Glutamate

This spice, produced by fermentation of beet sugar molasses, is ubiquitous in any Chinese kitchen "worth its salt." It has been associated with the Chinese Restaurant Syndrome characterized by itching, sweating, and sometimes headaches and feelings of great sleepiness. The last effect might be due to the glutamate, which can revert to glutamic acid in the body. Glutamic acid is an amino acid that acts on the brain as a chemical messenger, or neurotransmitter.

There has been increased concern about monosodium glutamate because some people develop a persistent depressive reaction for weeks after eating this spice. Most people who get sleepy or have other symptoms find that they fully recover within about eight hours. Another concern is that the glutamate releases sugar stores from the liver. This can cause the glucose reserves to be unavailable when needed.

Making the Dream Dreamier

There are some foods and food-drugs that make our dreams more bizarre. Opium eaters have been known to have fantastic dreams and Coleridge got ideas for "Kubla Khan" after taking opium. Thomas De Quincey, in his

Confessions of an English Opium Eater, reported marked changes in his dream life as he became addicted to opium.

LSD and other hallucinogens also seem to increase the fantasies of the dreamer. Although people who take them don't dream more, they do remember more. Morning glory seeds also have this effect. Some South American Indian cultures use the vine extract yage, which has hallucinogenic properties, because they feel that the dreams they have under the effects of this plant will foretell the future. Similar, though reduced, effects have been reported about magic mushrooms and cacti with power (especially mescal cactus).

What about cannabis and dreams? There have not been any detailed studies to date, but dream reports tend to be reliable. It is rare to find a user who reports fantastic dreams after eating or smoking marijuana. In fact, some users say that dreaming seems to counteract the effects of the weed-vegetable. Since there are many varieties of cannabis with different chemical compositions, research is necessary to verify sleep and dream effects.

Survey Results

In a recent survey, I asked two hundred people to list those foods that have discernible effects upon them, and to describe the effects. Some of the findings were surprising. Thirty-six responded that eating red meats made them lethargic or sleepy. Another twelve reported that red meats made them feel sedentary or sluggish.

Almost forty respondents reported that milk made them sleepy, although fourteen indicated that it made them relaxed and content. Camomile tea made six people sleepy and fourteen said that eating potatoes made them sleepy or drowsy. Sixteen reported that foods high in fats made them feel tired and rundown, lazy, drowsy, or sleepy. Ten reported that beer made them feel that way and six said pasta had that effect. Turkey was singled out by six people as a sleep-producing meat. Surprisingly, six people also reported that sugar made them sleepy, although some remarked that the first effect was stimulating. Six people also said that white bread made them sleepy.

Insomnia Foods

Certain foods tend to offset sleep. We earlier mentioned Chianti wine, aged cheese, and pickled herring. Coffee, tea, chocolate, and cola beverages deter sleep in many and make it less productive in some.

Plants such as the ephedra, source of ephedrine, act to reduce sleep. The coca leaf, source of cocaine and similar alkaloids, and khat, a vegetable widely eaten in Yemen and termed the cocaine of Africa, act in the same way.

Plants with the belladonna alkaloids (e.g., jimson weed, potato and tomato leaves) offset sleep, although those containing scopolamine will induce the so-called twilight amnesiac sleep—but this is far from natural sleep.

Foods made with stimulant herbs and spices such as saffron, borage, and nutmeg will tend to keep the night lights burning.

Asynchrony and Foods—
Seeking Drugs to Find a Rhythm

Asynchrony occurs when a person's internal rhythms are at odds with the demands of his environment. For example, some night workers' bodies say "sleep" while their jobs say "Awake!" This results in their feeling out of tune. In fact, this was one of the big complaints of the Colonists against King George III. The Declaration of Independence says, "... He has called together legislative bodies at places unusual, uncomfortable and distant for the sole purpose of fatiguing them." One important result of asynchrony in our time is the dependence of many people on food-drugs.

There are clearly "night people" and "day people." A night person is not ready for work or companionship early in the morning. Winston Churchill was famous as a late sleeper. When asked if he breakfasted with his wife he replied, "My wife and I tried two or three times in the last forty years to have breakfast together, but it was so disagreeable we had to stop."

It is unfortunate that many people must awaken much too early for their bodies, which want to sleep, and then stay awake late at night feeling good. Even if these people went to sleep earlier, their sleep would be of poor quality. As a result, people in asynchrony seek stimulants such as coffee and tea in the morning to awaken their body faster, then use depressants at night to help them sleep. It is a sad situation because if left to their own rhythms, they would probably be much more productive and certainly happier. Life in modern society has been devised by the early riser.

Moreover, many people feel that during a creative time, more sleep is essential. During a managerial or production phase, they need less. However, our industrialized society with its highly scheduled hours tends to ignore individual variables.

The problem becomes one of drug use (food-drugs and others) to maintain function. Perhaps people should begin examining their personal cycles and activity clocks during their high school and college years, and choose jobs compatible with their rhythms.

Sleep Disorders and Treatment with Foods

Narcolepsy

This is a condition characterized by frequent falling asleep during the normal waking period. A person with this condition may seem to nod off even during conversation.

The sleep lasts for only a few seconds or at most a few minutes but it is very disturbing to the narcoleptic.

People with this condition should avoid foods containing tryptophan and keep to low-protein foods during the day. Use of caffeine beverages and stimulant cheeses may counteract this tendency enough to reduce the need for stimulant drugs. Tea made from the ephedra plant may also help.

Nightmares

These are hard to avoid, although eating before sleep may precipitate them. The Indian plant snakeroot can help temporarily since it reduces the incidence of dreaming. It contains reserpine and other alkaloids, and actually was the forerunner of many potent tranquilizing medicines in current use.

The Pickwickian

Some obese people are always falling asleep. The condition is associated with the retention of large amounts of carbon dioxide, which has a narcotizing effect. The name comes from one of the characters in Dickens's *The Pickwick Papers* who was quite obese and somnolent. The food cure for this condition may be *no food,* which will result in weight loss and resolution of the problem. A trial of a few days of complete fasting will show whether this problem can be reduced through a diet. Certainly such a weight reduction diet should be carefully chosen to reduce choline, lecithin, and tryptophan.

Calcium

The sleepiest salt seems to be the one with calcium. Excessively low levels of calcium result in great increases in excitability of the brain and the muscles. The slightest tap will often cause muscle twitches. On the other hand, excessive levels of calcium result in great lethargy and hypersomnolence (sleeping all the time).

At normal levels calcium keeps the brain and muscles stable. It is important to maintain a good calcium intake particularly in the winter, since sunshine helps the body synthesize vitamin D and aids in the absorption of calcium. Vitamin D supplements are not usually needed since milk has added vitamin D. Beware of beans and peas—the phytic acid they contain taken together with calcium will result in a chemical reaction making calcium unavailable for the body. Herbalists consider calcium most important in sleep.

When calcium is infused into the brain fluid of experimental animals, sleep results. Because of the slow passage of substances between the brain and the blood, and the controls on the salts of the brain that keep it the most stable area of the body, it is unlikely that a single meal high in calcium will have much effect. On the other hand, a continued intake of adequate calcium may result in a level slightly higher than normal, with a resultant tendency toward overall tranquility. This is far from being proven, however.

Calcium sources include milk and dairy products, bone meal, green vegetables, meats, and soybeans.

Herbs

Some plants have been so potent in inducing sleep that medicines have been derived from them. Certainly we are all aware of the opium poppy whose very name, *Papaver somniferum* ("sleep-bearing poppy"), shows its effects. The henbane plant, from which the alkaloid scopolamine is derived, has been used to induce sleep for many centuries. Even Socrates was aware of the henbane, as were witches through the ages. Valerian, from the roots of the *Valeriana officinalis,* has been known as a sedative for thousands of years owing to its alkaloids, particularly chatinine.

Tiring Teas

While the tea made from *Thea sinensis* is essentially a stimulant and in larger amounts produces a pleasant altered state of awareness as well as tranquility, some teas made from other plants have sleep-inducing effects. Valerian is a particularly sleepy tea.

Catnip tea from the plant *Nepeta cataria,* a member of the mint family, produces mild sedation and a feeling of well-being. This plant is available at pet stores, sold for the pleasure and tranquility it causes in cats. Its active substance is called nepetalactone.

The hops plant, used in beer manufacturing, also produces a satisfying, tranquilizing tea.

Fatiguing Flowers

Narcissus fell in love with his reflection and subsequently pined away. He was turned into a flower bearing his name. Perhaps his pining away came from an overdose of the narcissus, which can be a potent sleep inducer and, in larger doses, a cause of altered consciousness. This quality comes from a substance that inhibits cholinesterase, the body chemical that breaks down acetylcholine. Acetylcholine is involved with sleep and dreaming and, in small doses, is safe. In larger doses, acetylcholine can induce paralysis.

The yellow marigold may also produce sleepiness. Many people eat marigolds indirectly and often. The bright yellow color seen in the skin of some chickens—particularly well-selling ones—is thought to indicate a healthy, fatty bird. However, this yellow color may actually come from feeding the chicken marigold petals. When we eat the chicken, we also eat some of the marigold.

Magnesium

The trace metal magnesium seems also to be important in sleep. Alcoholics may have reduced amounts of magnesium, contributing to their frequent sleep disorders. Magnesium has been used medically as an anticonvulsant because of its quieting effect upon the brain. Since it is so widely dispersed in foods, deficiencies are unlikely to occur. In some cases of severe or prolonged diarrhea, however, the magnesium level might fall and result in sleep disorders. With prolonged fasting, sleep disturbances may be aggravated by magnesium deficiency. Magnesium is found in meats, milk, and leafy vegetables grown in soil containing magnesium.

Lobster

Lobster has a high concentration of gamma amino butyric acid, which is known to be an inhibitory transmitter of the brain. If anyone can afford a diet high in lobster, he will probably experience some sleepiness. For the alert lobster lover, sleepiness is a small price to pay for a high-priced lobster.

Food Additives

We know that monosodium glutamate can make us sleepy. An interesting finding, reported in the *Tokyo Science Journal* in December 1964, was that sodium propionate can induce paradoxical sleep (like dreaming sleep) in the cat. Sensitive people may find their white bread, to which sodium propionate has been added, to be a staff of sleepy life. In my study of two hundred people, six reported that white bread made them drowsy. Whether this was due to the wheat used or an additive is uncertain. Dr. Claude Frazier, a renowned allergist, noted (in 1978) that certain people seem to be sensitive to wheat and white bread, with resultant feelings of lassitude.

Emulsifiers

Many foods contain lecithin, which is added as an emulsifier to enable fats to mix well and not separate—

mayonnaise is an example. This fatty substance is ordinarily made in the body from orally ingested choline. Recent research has demonstrated that lecithin directly affects the production of acetylcholine in the brain. Because acetylcholine has been implicated in sleep mechanisms, it is possible that lecithin will cause drowsiness. Certainly high-fat diets tend to produce fatigue and sleepiness. In fact, sixteen people out of my sample of two hundred reported this effect from high fats.

The Lithium Salt

One psychiatric illness is called "manic-depressive" psychosis. People in mania speak constantly, are constantly in motion, and have thoughts that fly from one subject to the next. They sleep little in such a state. Scientific studies over the past thirty years have shown how lithium salts can be extremely effective in bringing such people to normalcy. Nathan Kline, M.D., a well-known psychiatrist and expert on this condition, has speculated that high lithium content in the water and soil of certain areas may reduce the frequency of this psychosis. One of the first signs of response in a "manic" patient is a return to regular sleep patterns.

The best foods for lithium are those from the oceans, or those grown in soil with a high lithium content. A recent (1978) report in the *New England Journal of Medicine* by William Millington along with Dr. Anthony McCall and Dr. Richard Wurtman suggests that such patients can be aided even more by increasing the choline in the diet. Thus a calming diet would include both choline and lithium-rich foods. On the other hand, an anti-depressant diet (for a fatigued, apathetic, depressed person) should have *reduced* choline as an important basis.

7 Foods for Creativity

The Romans saw the forces of inspiration that led to creation and beauty. They saw, too, the exalted state that was part of the creative act. To explain what was happening, they developed the idea of a genius. The genius, not to be confused with modern ideas of genius, was a spirit that resided within each person and, when awakened, was the source of creative inspiration. Each place also had its genius which watched over it.

Creativity and religious experiences seem related, both being associated with an external impulse or inspiration arising (an idea "came to me"). Both are associated with "seeing the light" and with some altered states of consciousness. The holy kabbala, the ancient Jewish mystical doctrine, includes creativity as one of the paths of wisdom and gates of true understanding of the nature of God. It tells us that the "illumined intelligence" is a goal toward which we must strive. Though the creative state is more than illumination because it has a vital component, the illumination is translated into deed—the word is made flesh.

The psychoanalyst Ernst Kris, who spent much of his career fascinated by the phenomenon of creativity, said, "In inspiration, the individual is driven. He is in an exceptional stage. Thoughts and images tend to flow, things appear in his mind of which he never seemed to have known."

The act of creation does involve opening gates of the mind with a feeling of great exhilaration, although during a creative process a person may experience rapid mood changes, and be extremely emotional.

Foods, drugs, and beverages are intimately associated with the creative process. Those foods that assist in removing the veil of day-to-day functioning to allow for "letting go" set the stage for inspiration and originality to emerge.

Creativity Stimulants

Certainly alcohol and other fermented beverages have played a prominent role, probably by quieting the usual inhibitions. William Faulkner said that he couldn't begin writing without a bottle of Scotch nearby. Ernest Hemingway and F. Scott Fitzgerald used alcohol to help open their creative gates, as have many other writers.

Henri Poincaré, the brilliant mathematician, found that coffee was useful for him. He said that after coffee, "Ideas arose in crowds. I felt them collide until pairs interlocked."

Baudelaire and other writers found that hashish would be stimulatory. For Coleridge, the dreams produced from taking opium were inspiring.

Rimbaud discovered that absinthe had powerful effects that stimulated his inspiration. Derived from the wormwood plant, real absinthe has been outlawed in this country due to its addicting qualities. An unusual chemical, thujone, is in fairly high concentration in true absinthe. It is still used as a flavoring in vermouth, but in small amounts. Thujone is a major component of cedar leaf oil and is present in significant amounts in sage. Chemically it is similar to nutmeg.

Writers often use a variety of stimulants to get them

started. When asked about his writing habits James Jones (best known for his novel *From Here to Eternity*) said, "After I get up it takes me an hour and a half of fiddling around before I can get up the courage and nerve to work. I smoke half a pack of cigarettes, drink six or seven cups of coffee and read over what I did the day before. Finally I go to the typewriter."

William Burroughs was in South America when he tried a plant called yage which, as he said, "gave me a lot of copy."

Aldous Huxley used the peyote cactus, and the psychologist Havelock Ellis also gained inspiration from mescaline. Weir Mitchell, an endocrinologist, claimed to enhance his perception of the complex interrelation of the hormones through the use of mescaline.

A. E. Housman found beer to be conducive to poetic thoughts. He was also a tea drinker and once made the remark that when he was having difficulty completing a poem, "a third stanza came with a little coaxing after tea." W. H. Auden made the comment that while writing, "I drink endless cups of tea."

Walter de la Mare said he had to have nicotine from smoking to be able to write, and Stephen Spender used cigarettes as well as coffee. Hemingway used alcohol, coffee, and cigarettes, and eventually succumbed to lung cancer, probably as a result of his heavy smoking.

Freud used cocaine for years. Its sensual, stimulating effects may well have played a role in his concern with sexuality in the mental processes.

Cocaine has been used by many well-known authors. Arthur Conan Doyle, the creator of Sherlock Holmes, used it, as did Holmes in the novels. Robert Louis Stevenson used cocaine, and Dr. Jekyll and Mr. Hyde have been seen as an illustration of the effects of overdosage. Today, multiple stimulants are often used. For example, it is not uncommon for coffee, tea, cocaine, marijuana, nicotine, wine, and spirits to be consumed within a period of several hours. The major danger of these combinations results from a hyperexcitability of the heart. Deaths have been reported from such a combination.

There seem to be four basic types of food-drugs used to enhance creativity. First, there are stimulants such as coffee, tea, cocaine, and chocolate. The second group are the stimulants that cause distinctly altered states of consciousness—mescaline, psilocybin mushrooms, absinthe (with thujone), and possibly to a lesser extent, LSD. The third type includes mild depressants such as alcoholic beverages which seem to relieve inhibitions. The fourth group induces mixed stimulant-depressant effects—red wines, cigarettes, etc.

Large Meals and the Creative Letdown

Large meals and the intemperate use of food seem to act against creative impulses. I was unable to find any notable who found a large meal helpful, although Mozart supposedly was inspired after a meal—but only after taking exercise.

Perhaps the old cliché that the creative artist has to be hungry to produce his best work has basis in fact as well as finances. Certainly during a storm of creative impulses thoughts of food seem to be dispelled. Perhaps it is because the creative experience is so overpowering that the usual drives are subordinated to it. The work may become like food and is often spoken of in food terms. For example, Mozart said that when writing his music, "It soon occurs to me how I may turn on this or that morsel to act so as to make a good dish of it." A. E. Housman likened poetry to that of an internal secretion of the body. Thomas Wolfe said, "There is a quality of intemperate excess—an almost insane hunger to devour the entire body of human experience."

Fasting seems to induce an altered state of consciousness for creative inspiration and introspection. This has been realized by religions throughout the world, and almost all of them include some fasting as part of their ceremonies. This has been carried to extremes—for example, an Inca prince who was going to become the chief priest of Peru reportedly had to fast for a month before assuming his role.

In a creative state, however, decreased eating is self-imposed. It seems that the initial push for the creative process may come from particular foods and drugs that help to induce the desired consciousness. But once the creative energy is started, eating becomes secondary. Thus, van Gogh would awaken and almost immediately become lost in his work, not stopping to eat for many hours.

Vitamins for Creation

The diminished eating associated with the creative act will ordinarily exert no untoward effects because the body has built up prior stores, particularly of the B vitamins. It is interesting that mental anomalies, retardation, and depressions are common results of B-vitamin deficiency. However, supplemental vitamins should probably not be taken during the creative act since it might upset a delicate balance. Before beginning a book, painting, or other creative project, a person should maintain good nutrition and take supplemental B and C vitamins—no difficulty should then be experienced even if food is deficient for several weeks. Competitive sports during a creative period are probably detrimental.

Lessons from Charlie Chaplin

Many creative people find that the need for a certain food or drink as an adjunct to their art becomes almost obsessional. We humans exhibit what are called state-bound feelings.

In the film *City Lights,* Charlie Chaplin prevents a drunken millionaire from committing suicide and becomes his savior and friend. However, a problem arises. When sober, the millionaire doesn't recognize Charlie anymore and boots him out of his house. Fortunately for Charlie the millionaire doesn't remain sober for long, and when drunk again recognizes Charlie and welcomes him warmly. The lesson here is that the memory and feelings tend to become state-bound. Material learned during a particular state can best be remembered when there is a return to the same state. Realists recognize this sort of problem even in interpersonal relations. For example, a man who falls in love with a woman during an altered state of consciousness may have to return to that altered state to recapture the feeling.

An artist who awakens his genius with alcohol—or the smell of rotten apples—finds that he must return to that stimulus to again feel the mood of creativity. Faulkner could not write without his Scotch handy. Because he might have gained inspiration and a feeling of where his novel was going and felt the excitement of creation while under the influence of alcohol, in order to get back to those thoughts and feelings he would have to consume alcohol again.

An account of a simple experiment by Dr. D. W. Goodwin published in *Science* in 1969 clearly demonstrated this state-related aspect of learning. He had forty-eight subjects memorize nonsense syllables while drunk. When sober they had a great deal of difficulty remembering what they had learned. However, when they were given alcohol again, their memory remarkably returned.

It's possible that this might relate to a student studying for a test. If, for example, the student fasted during his learning he might have better recall if he took his test while fasting.

Similarly, the insights experienced while under the influence of a hallucinogenic plant are recalled better when in that state again. This may also account for recurrent dreams where we know we dreamed the same thing but do not remember the content.

Perhaps this state-relatedness helps us categorize experiences for recall or return. Many of us know that it is difficult to work away from the regular desk or setting. For creativity, this can be worth remembering. If a food or state has been associated with creative flashes, a return to the setting and state induced by food or drink may be helpful in reawakening similar flashes. Marcel Proust demonstrated such flashes when he wrote, ". . . One day in winter, as I came home, my mother, seeing that I was cold, offered me some tea, a thing I did not ordinarily take. . . . I raised to my lips a spoonful of the tea in which I had soaked a morsel of the cake. No sooner had the warm liquid, and the crumbs with it, touched my palate than a shudder ran through my whole body. . . . And suddenly the memory all returns." And then he wrote *Swann's Way*.

CREATIVITY STIMULANTS

Alcohol
Coffee
Tea
Beer
Absinthe
Cocaine
Yage
Peyote
Psilocybin mushrooms

Chocolate
Wine
Betel nuts
Opium
Cannabis
Cola beverages
Tobacco
Fasting

Foods for Sexuality, Reproduction, and Gland Stimulation

8

Our human society is unique in the animal kingdom. It is the only one where the female can be ready for sex every day.

Sexuality is used not only for reproduction, but for entertainment and relaxation. Now that birth control pills and a variety of other birth control techniques are so widely used, and with a decreasing societal inhibition on the flowering of women's sexuality, sex for its own sake (closeness, release, entertainment, relaxation, etc.) seems to be the rule rather than the exception.

The influences upon sexuality are diverse and complex. Some foods have long been prized for their aphrodisiac effects and while some claims are clearly fanciful, others have a basis in scientific fact. A brief description of sexual chemistry is important in understanding food and drug effects.

The marked influence the brain can have is seen in a variety of brain diseases that may be associated with hypersexuality. Artificial stimulation by electric current of animal brains has elicited mating behavior and profound changes in sexual interest. Certain brain stimulation will produce penile erection in male animals. This assumes importance because some foods tend to heighten sexual interest in men. To further demonstrate that brain mechanisms have a role in male erection there is the unexplained phenomenon that approximately 80 percent of the rapid eye movement (REM) periods during sleep (associated with dreaming) are accompanied by erection in the male.

The cerebral cortex (the most advanced part of the brain) seems to be necessary for sexual behavior in men, although all aspects of reproduction can occur in a female in the absence of a cerebral cortex—all, of course, except for awareness and pleasure. The fact that the cerebral cortex is so closely involved with male sexuality relates to the inhibition many men experience from psychological stresses, and the inhibition of male capability with depressants such as alcohol.

More primitive portions of the brain are also closely associated with sexual behavior, desire, and performance. The limbic system, thought by many to be involved with emotional responses, and the primitive olfactory area, having to do with the sense of smell, are both associated. Smell can still be a powerful sexual stimulant although its importance has decreased in the last few thousand years. Still, foods that either enhance or do not diminish smell can be stimulators in some people. Since taste and smell are often bound together, spicy and pungent foods have historically been associated with heightened sexuality. Some of these stimulate the nervous system as well—for example, pepper, nutmeg, cubeb (Java pepper), and saffron.

Gland functions are intimately related to sexual development and function. The pineal gland, the "inner eye" of man, is a mysterious organ although it definitely is involved in the age at which maturation occurs. The use of light to stimulate a pineal hormone, melatonin, inhibits sexual development—a factor that points to a dimly lit setting as being more conducive to sexuality.

The hypothalamus is a portion of the brain seen as a

controller of many responses. The pituitary, also called the master gland, a pea-sized, unimportant-looking but vital structure, sits right below the hypothalamus. The pituitary gland secretes many hormones involved directly or indirectly with sexual activities including female menstrual cycles, male formation of sperm, and production of male hormones.

The thyroid gland controls the metabolism of the body and is involved with sexual activity as well as fertility. One of the symptoms of decreased thyroid function is loss of sexual desire; people who begin taking thyroid hormone often report an increase in sexual interest. Some foods with antithyroid substances, such as turnips, kale, cabbage, and soybeans, may inhibit sexuality when eaten as a constant and relatively large part of the diet.

The adrenal cortex secretes not only cortisone but also other hormones that influence sexual development and drive. Patients taking cortisone for medical conditions often experience a marked enhancement of sexual urges. Some foods contain cortisonelike compounds which might account for their sex-stimulating actions—sarsaparilla and ginseng are examples.

Hormonal production requires adequate nutritional building blocks. Foods containing male hormone structures (e.g., testes of chicken or turkey) can add some hormonal building blocks for men. Foods with estrogen effects can similarly act to supplement deficiencies in women. Such foods as yams, hops, palm kernels, pomegranate seeds, and carrots (and their seeds) have estrogen factors. Others will be described later in this chapter.

Casanova was a great popularizer of oysters—this renowned lover reportedly ate fifty oysters every evening. Could it have done the trick for him? There is a scientific basis for Casanova's claims. In the first place, oysters in this quantity are a good source of protein. But even more to the point, the oyster is a rich source of iodine, an element necessary for proper functioning of the thyroid gland. A deficient thyroid can cause lidibo to fade away and an active (though not overactive) thyroid keeps the glands moving and the whole body running smoothly. Other iodine-rich foods such as seaweed and fish also act in a stimulatory manner.

As if this were not enough, a recent conference dealing with foods from the sea and some new books about marine foods demonstrate that sterols are present in oysters and other mollusks. A sterol is a chemical form of the same configuration as sex hormones and cortisone. And zinc, an important trace metal, is high in oysters.

Importance of High Protein

Many of the sexual secretions contain protein. The building blocks of protein, the amino acids, must be present in sufficient quantity for efficient glandular function. Many hormones are composed of various amino acids linked together. For example, thyroid hormone comes from action of iodine on the amino acid tyrosine, which is found in heavy amounts in red meats and milk. Fasting will reduce thyroid hormone—a logical adaptation that slows metabolism and conserves calories in a state of deficient food.

The hypothalamic substances that stimulate production and release of pituitary hormones, and other chemical messengers that stimulate hormones are composed of amino acids. Just imagine the effects of a prolonged diet without protein—wasting, hormone deficiencies, apathy, mental impairments, and a sexual urge that went away after a few days. It is not just coincidence that prisoners of war kept on deficient diets for weeks, months, or years reported that they had little thought of sex, although there were certainly many other stresses. Those on fasts report reduced sex drive after the first few days, and studies have verified that fasting will reduce thyroid function and function of the sympathetic nervous system, which has to do with sexual arousal. A patient of mine who had contracted a venereal disease on one of his out-of-town trips and did not want to repeat his experience discovered that complete fasting reduced his sexual drives.

It is logical that our sex drive would go down when not enough protein or protein of the wrong amino acid type is eaten—secretions of the body and chemical processes needing protein cannot be made without protein. Looking at our evolutionary history, men and women would be expected to have increased sex drive and reproducing ability with a high-protein diet. A period when the hunt is good and there is ample food would certainly be a better time to have offspring than during a famine when the children would be an additional burden and would tend to be sickly.

When the protein intake decreases, the secretion of the principal male hormone is decreased. Similarly, less estrogen and progesterone are secreted. It often has been noted that under conditions of hardship women's menstrual periods cease or become irregular.

A purely vegetarian diet tends to decrease sexual drive in men since certain proteins and amino acids are in lesser quantities. Such a diet may tend to induce a more relaxed state, with decreased aggressive drives and a more contemplative attitude. This sort of diet tends to have less choline, which is found in highest quantities in egg yolks and meat. It goes into the formation of acetylcholine, the active transmitter of the parasympathetic nervous system, which has much to do with males attaining erection and with the production of sexual secretions.

The reduction of sexuality with a strict vegetarian diet makes good sense if interpersonal nonsexual interactions are desired. For example, at the Living Love Center in Berkeley, California, some of the seminars are held with participants wearing no clothes. The complete vegetarian diets followed there enable such relating with less interference from primitive sexual drives. Buddhists and members of other sects or religions seeking desire-free states usually have vegetarianism as their dietary norm.

Sensual Vegetables

Carrots

The carrot contains the vitamin-A-forming substance carotene, which is a steroidlike substance and also figures in hormone-making actions of the adrenal cortex. Vitamin A is important for vision and overall brain activity.

Carrot seed extract contains a hormonelike substance that is reported to exert an effect like that of birth control pills. The Greeks considered carrots to be aphrodisiacs, and with the vitamin A content and the hormonelike substance of the seeds, there is some basis for their belief.

Sarsaparilla

There is an image of aging men in the old West drinking a brew of sarsaparilla (the root of the smilax bush) to regain potency. On analysis, this tea contains steroid compounds similar to the structure of the sex hormones progesterone and testosterone. Where is the sarsaparilla of our life? Technology is taking away some potent plants and substituting artificial flavors and colors in their places—sarsaparilla is one example.

Ginseng

As in the old-time medicine show, ginseng could be billed as "snake oil—good for what ails you" because of its widespread use for a myriad of conditions. Usually advertised as an aid to male potency, this Oriental herb has found its way into the pharmacies of America. Not surprisingly, I saw ginseng in many drugstores in California. However, upon finding ginseng in the small town of Lumberton, New Jersey, I knew how far this herb had spread. The current interest in America is a resurgence rather than a new addition. In Colonial America ginseng was cultivated and even exported in large quantities. William Byrd wrote in 1738, "The Earth has never produced any vegetable so friendly to man as Ginseng. Nor do I say this at random, or by the strength of my faith, but by my own experience. I have found it very cordial and reviving after great fatigue, it warms the blood, frisks the spirits, strengthens the stomach and comforts the bowels exceedingly. All this it performs without any of those naughty effects that might make men too troublesome and impertinent to their poor wives."

Ginseng is the root of a plant called *Panax ginseng* which grows in China and Korea. It is an important drug in Oriental medicine and has been used as a tonic and rejuvenator. In ancient China, ginseng was called the "King of Herbs" and was felt to aid longevity. The U.S. production of ginseng is also high. In fact, according to *The New York Times*, ginseng exports in 1977 were valued at a record 26.5 million dollars. Now, with increased China–U.S. interaction, scientists in both countries have renewed interest in studying this unusual vegetable.

Despite its widespread usage there is no information about ginseng in the latest edition of the authoritative medical work dealing with drugs and medicines (L. S. Goodman and A. Gilman, *The Pharmacological Basis of Therapeutics*). To paraphrase Hamlet, "All is not contained within your philosophy, Horatio."

Ginseng, however, has been the subject of many scientific papers since it has been reported by many people to increase work capacity as well as nonspecific responses to stress. Treatment of rats with ginseng stepped up their ability to withstand heat stresses and seemed to stimulate their adrenal glands. Russian scientific literature has some brief references to work attempting to evaluate the effects of ginseng on the longevity of mice, but since it is available to American readers only in abstract form it is difficult to evaluate.

American writers have confirmed that ginseng seems to have a general, mildly beneficial influence on the body's stress mechanism and decreases strain on body glands, particularly the adrenal. Hans Selye, one of the world's leading experts on the subject of stress, spends two pages in his cumulative medical work, *Stress in Health and Disease*, summarizing scientific studies on ginseng, most of which appear to support the reported benefits.

Despite the apparent lack of attention to ginseng in our country, Anthony Huxley, author of *Plant and Planet*, reports that a Japanese company has built a plant to produce saponins, from which estrogens are made, using special growth techniques on ginseng.

The Coca Leaf and Sex

The coca vegetable, source of cocaine and many other compounds, is chewed by the Indians of Peru, who live at high altitudes. When chewed with ash which releases the alkaloids, it markedly enhances work capacity and ability to tolerate low oxygen. In addition, coca is a vitamin-rich food—important because it also reduces the appetite. Dr. Andrew Weil, director of the Harvard Botanical Museum, has written of how it is used to supplement the diet with needed vitamins and minerals, particularly in some nutritionally deficient areas of South America.

Freud became interested in cocaine in the early 1880s and found that the drug gave him good feelings and aided him in his periods of melancholy. His interest was so great that by 1884 he had written a paper called "Über Coca" which was published in Germany and in December 1884 in *The Saint Louis Medical and Surgical Journal*. This paper, showing Freud's self-experimentation with the coca leaf and cocaine as well as his detailed knowledge of the drug, is a remarkable study—as up-to-date now as when it was written. Perhaps Freud had a lot of initial enthusiasm about the benefits of cocaine because he dealt with it carefully and did not foresee the consequences of prolonged excessive use. Freud's interests gradually shifted, and another paper in 1885 further detailed the effects of cocaine with a mention of its aphrodisiac qualities.

Though Freud gradually backed away from his position of the harmlessness of cocaine, he continued using it himself particularly while writing one of his essential works, *The Interpretation of Dreams*. He wrote in a letter to his fiancée, Martha Bernays, in 1884, "Woe to you, my princess, when I come, I will kiss you quite red and feed you till you are plump. And if you are forward you shall see who is the stronger, a gentle little girl who doesn't eat enough or a big wild man who has cocaine in his body. In my last severe depression, I took coca again and a small dose lifted me to the heights in a wonderful fashion . . ."

In "Über Coca," Freud said the Peruvian Indian uses the coca leaf "when he is faced with a difficult journey, when he takes a woman, or in general whenever his strength is taxed he increases his usual dose."

The belief of the natives of South America in the sexually stimulating effects of cocaine is attested to by their depiction of their goddess of love with coca leaves in her hand. South Americans also feel that cocaine can restore or allow retention of potency in men well into old age. In "Über Coca" Freud said, "Among the persons to whom I have given coca, three reported violent sexual excitement which they unhesitatingly attributed to the coca."

In the 1880s Parke, Davis and Company, then a small firm, prepared pure cocaine. In discussing its therapeutic indications, the company cited use as a stimulant, for gastric disorders, for cachexia, as an anesthetic, and as an aphrodisiac.

While use of coca is illegal in our country except in medicines, those who obtain the drug illegally confirm the effects upon sexuality. In my clinical experience, one patient being treated for a sudden nose bleed, with cocaine packing as anesthesia, mentioned to me his sudden sexual heightening.

As an aphrodisiac, cocaine probably played a substantial role in the formulation of Freud's theories. In that time of inhibited sexual activity, with his fiancée living far away and with his use of cocaine, it seems reasonable to assume that Freud had a heightened sex drive with relatively few avenues of gratification. Being in touch with his heightened sexuality enabled him to write about it and no doubt he found that he could dissipate some of his sexual energies through his work, a process called sublimation in current psychoanalytic circles.

It is possible that the pure extract of cocaine is far more dangerous than the coca vegetable, which contains a variety, and possibly a good balance, of vitamins and stimulants. The Peruvian Indians chew it daily for years with no apparent adverse effects.

Other Plants for Sexual Power

In Chinese medicine, the ephedra plant was used for a variety of purposes. We now use the product of the plant, ephedrine, to keep the airways open in asthma. A commonly reported side effect is increased sexuality. A similar effect has been found with a plant called *Catha edulis* which is chewed by most adults in Yemen. Tea made with this plant, which grows wild in Nevada and other areas in the West, has carried the nickname "whorehouse tea" for at least one hundred years.

Marijuana and Sex

No scientific study has been done concerning the effects of marijuana upon sexuality. Dr. Harris Rubin, a researcher at the University of Southern Illinois School of Medicine, had a government research grant to study this subject, but at the last minute funds were withdrawn.

There is a good deal of confusion on this topic. One report seemed to show that men who were frequent users had lower testosterone levels, but subsequent reports were contradictory. There are no definite scientific answers, but user reports are generally consistent. The smoke from the cannabis plant and the tea made from the leaves produces feelings of contentment and well-being. In addition, older medical works (for example, *Potter's Therapeutics, Materia Medica and Pharmacy,* 1926) considers cannabis to be a "powerful aphrodisiac."

Cooking with marijuana is becoming more common— not only is it used in marijuana brownies, but in stews, casseroles, etc. Commonly the plant is first boiled in water and butter for several hours and is then strained. After cooling, the green butter rises to the top and solidifies. This is then used in many recipes. After eating marijuana, men generally report enhanced sexual pleasure, although with large amounts some report difficulty in getting an erection. For women it seems to have aphrodisiac qualities.

One survey of twenty women demonstrated that all found marijuana use stimulated their sexual drive—provided the setting and partner were appropriate. If they were not appropriate, it acted in the opposite way. Many contradictory findings about marijuana may be explained by considering it to be a mood intensifier. Another reason for contradictory reports doubtless relates to the type and amount of active substances present—these may vary considerably depending on farming techniques, seeds, sunlight, and duration of storage. As with any vegetable, agricultural techniques are an important, although sometimes inadequately considered, factor in terms of chemical composition. As illustrated in chapter 3, vitamins can vary tremendously depending on sunlight.

If a woman feels sensual, then she may become sexier with this herb. As in Proverbs 15:17, "Better is a dinner of herbs where love is . . ."

Vitamins: Which, When, and How Much?

There is no question that adequate vitamins are needed for sexual functioning in men and women. But which can really help? Which need replacement in a person whose sexual life is one of kaleidoscopic vigor? These questions may not have definite answers. A true deficiency of a vitamin or vitamins can result in inadequate sexual function. To assume the converse is incorrect logic—i.e., if a deficiency causes problems, an excess cannot be assumed to produce super potency. But a brief mention of vitamins is worthwhile.

VITAMIN A: People need vitamin A to produce the sexual secretions. However, deficiencies would be unlikely in those with a normal diet.

VITAMIN B: This group is needed for glandular and pituitary function. Deficiencies of vitamin B_6 and vitamin B_{12} can cause sexual impairment.

VITAMIN C: That oft-discussed ascorbic acid and source of fervent scientific debate is no doubt related to hormone synthesis and body tissue repair. There is little evidence that supplementation has any effects upon sexuality. However, there might be beneficial effects in the female resulting from acidification of the vaginal area and a lesser tendency for fungus or yeast infections.

VITAMIN E: This vitamin is in vogue for a variety of reasons. The original work demonstrated that deficiency of vitamin E in rats causes atrophy of the male tubules through which the sperm flows, as well as decreased sperm formation. Little or no effect has yet been demonstrated in man, but since seeds, a good source of vitamin E, are also a good source of sterol-like substances that go into hormone makeup, perhaps the vitamin E exerts some effects. The door to new information about vitamin E is open.

Hormone Stews

Chicken giblets include testicles and ovaries as well as the heart and other organs. If the chickens have been bred well, have had a chance to use these organs, and if hormone supplements have not been given to them, these giblets should be separated and made into a "male" stew and a "female" stew. The hearts might be better in the "male" stew. Women might want to try both since small amounts of testosterone, the male hormone, may increase sex drive. The opposite (estrogens for men) might have the reverse effect. Chicken livers may be high in estrogenlike substances.

Plant foods with estrogenlike effects include hops, date seeds, pomegranate seeds, yams, and soybeans.

Chocolate—The Brown Devil

Francisco Carletti, a Spanish adventurer of the late 1500s, saw the Mexicans mix little chocolate cakes with water, shake the mixture until a froth came up, and gulp the drink down. He observed that "it gives admirable pleasure and satisfaction of the bodily nature, to which it gives strength, nourishment, and vigor in such a way that those who are accustomed to drinking it cannot remain robust without it even when they eat other substantial things. And they appear to diminish when they don't have that drink." He saw the stimulant power of chocolate as well as what happens when a stimulant is taken too often.

Continued use can result in a mild depressive state when it is withdrawn. There is a scientific term for this, but what it really means is that the wisdom of the body tries to keep things at an equilibrium. When stimulated, the body compensates, so a few weeks of abstinence are needed if a stimulant is withdrawn after prolonged use.

In thinking about foods as well as drugs, remember that there is no "free lunch"—our bodies tend to compensate for excesses in every area and seek a balance. But as with most things, chocolate can be a pleasant stimulant drug experience when used in moderation. So powerful has it been perceived, however, that in the 1700s the Spanish government, under pressure from the Church, banned chocolate, calling it "a drink of the devil."

Before going into why chocolate stimulates as it does, the wary reader should know that many substances like candy bars believed to contain chocolate do not. We should lament! Where is the chocolate of our lives? Like many other potent foods, chocolate is often replaced by artificial look-alikes and taste-alikes.

Chocolate is the extract from the seed of the evergreen *Theobroma cacao. Theobroma* means "food of the gods," which gives some idea of the reverence accorded to chocolate by the ancients. Its major stimulating substance is theobromine, an alkaloid similar to caffeine. The Aztecs so delighted in the taste and effects of chocolate that they thought their god Quetzalcoatl brought the cacao seeds to earth from Paradise.

Is it indeed an aphrodisiac? Montezuma drank chocolate in homage to the goddess of love. *The True History of the Conquest of the New Spain* by Bernal Díaz del Castillo relates that Montezuma always took a cup before going off to visit one of his wives. Certainly chocolate was powerful enough to serve as money in the markets of ancient Mexico. In Ecuador, the beans are called *pepe de oro* ("seeds of gold").

Further accounts of the sexual uses of chocolate include a treatise by Joan Fran Rauch who wrote of it in 1624 as "a violent inflamer of the passions." When soaked with ambergris, a secretion from the sperm whale, it was considered to be a powerful sexual stimulant in the court of Louis XV. Even the Marquis de Sade, known for his wild parties, served it. In fact a description of eating chocolate at one of his parties was followed by: "All at once the guests, both men and women, were seized with a burning sensation of lustful ardor." And Casanova, the oyster lover and not one to miss any possible sexual inducer, used chocolate as a love stimulant. More recently, *Cosmopolitan* considered chocolate to be among the top ten aphrodisiacs.

But chocolate is not what is used to be. Even true chocolate goes through much processing today, which undoubtedly alters it. But at many stores and food markets where coffee beans and vanilla beans are sold, you can still find cocoa beans which can be mixed and mashed with vanilla and sugar and added to milk or water. Also, at supermarkets, baking chocolate has a high content of true chocolate. As with all plants of power, the amount of active substance may vary widely, so you might have to try different stores and shipments if at first you can't discern any effects. The search may be worth the effort.

A Lesson from the Centenarians of the Andes

Dr. David Davies, of the gerontological unit at University College in London, has been studying some unusual people who live in the mountains of Ecuador. One of their striking traits is their longevity. There are many people with documented ages of more than 100 years, and some above 125 years of age.

Passion and lovemaking are very important to this isolated community and there is no concept of a "dirty old man" or a "sexy old woman." Irrespective of age there is a lot of sexual activity with the women making overt advances as often as the men. Some men above 100 years of age still have frequent sexual relations, and men over 80 like to boast about the number of lovers they can take in a night.

One of the vegetable foods used by the men is believed to help them retain potency and sex drive. While the men were aided, use of the plant apparently diminished the women's drive. This plant, guarana, was mentioned by Dr. Davies, but he did not know its components.

Guarana is composed chiefly of the seeds of *Paullinia cupana*. Its ingredients include alkaloids, the principal one being caffeine; it also contains substances that make up a structural base for adrenalin, and very small amounts of hormonelike substances.

This plant seems to stimulate the sympathetic nervous system as do amphetamines and the ephedra plant, thereby stimulating the male sex drive. This goes along with the observations women have made that the latter two drugs produce too much nervousness, offsetting the calm that is helpful for a woman's best sexual state.

Another indication in this Ecuadorian community of the ongoing interest in sex is a small figurine representing an erect male penis that the women wear around their necks and the men carry in their pockets. This figure is generally small and carved out of stone for the women, larger and made of wood for the men.

In this society there is no fear that alcohol, drugs, or drink are injurious, and even those over 100 keep smoking and maintaining their other habits.

From this information it would be a mistake to conclude that guarana is a miracle drug, although its effects seem to warrant exploration, or that sexual vigor keeps people young. It can just as easily be that the interest in sex is a manifestation of the great vigor of these old people.

Several aspects of this society should be highlighted, however, even if their significance is unknown. The first is that there are documented records showing people living for more than 130 years. Men over 100 are potent, have active sperm, impregnate younger women, and generally retain a sharp and clear mind. According to Dr. Davies, women retain the ability to have children well into their fifties and often menstruation does not cease until sometime in the sixties.

As a physician, I find this startling. Dr. Louis Hellman, a renowned obstetrician and gynecologist who was my professor in medical school, challenged our class to find any woman in our culture who had given birth to a child when she was past the age of 50. We searched, one hundred eighty medical students looking for a childbearing woman beyond the age of 50. Nobody found one and now, twelve years later, I am still looking.

A Yam, What a Yam

Think of the Thanksgiving meal with a family gathered around the table preparing to eat their chemical feast. Yes, a chemical feast! For now let's focus on those yams filling the center dish—a traditional Thanksgiving delight. The yam, of the genus *Dioscorea,* originated, like Homo sapiens, in Africa. It has assumed much prominence as the most important food crop in Nigeria. Rural people along the Ivory Coast often subsist on a diet in which half of the calories come from the yam; in the African interior, the yam often makes up 25 percent of the diet.

But when the yam crop is good, thoughts go from using the yam as a food to using it in drugs. The yam has been used for centuries in Africa by witch doctors and neighborhood herbalists in the treatment of uterine and breast disorders as well as to reduce inflammation. It contains steroidlike substances similar to cortisone, and female sex hormones.

Originally cortisone and hormones such as estrogens were obtained from animal sources—a slow, painstaking, and expensive process. But using the yam requires a chemical process that is cheaper—and yams are readily available.

For a woman, the yam seems to be a source of a little extra hormone, benefits to the skin, and sexual secretions.

The yam, however, is not a total hormone success story, because it contains other components that deserve mentioning. Its phytic acid tends to bind calcium, making it unavailable for use by the body. Rickets (weak bones) are found frequently in underdeveloped countries where poverty forces the use of this food as too great a percentage of the diet.

The Japanese Turn-on

A fishy food prized as an aphrodisiac among the Japanese smart set is a dish called fugu. It is actually the puffer fish from the China Seas and its aphrodisiac effects come from a milky fluid secreted by the male fish's sex organs. It is served at many restaurants, and special chefs in Japan are trained in preparing it. However, overdosage produces a toxic effect on the spinal cord and death has even been reported. Overdosage is possible because there is no way to gauge just what quantity of active substance will be found. The female fish, not to be outdone, has tetrodotoxin in the ovaries, also a nerve toxin. Substances like these are similar to alcohol because of dose-related effects—a small dose pleasurable and a large one can be lethal. In cases of severe illness or death, the chef has his license revoked.

Fats and Femmes Fatales

The importance of fatty substances in sexual function relates to the lipids of the body. The ovaries contain large amounts of cholesterol and fatty acids, and a biochemical synthesis route for hormones begins with cholesterol. Those on a severely restricted fat diet may well experience decrease in sexual desire. In men the fatty acid content of the testes corresponds to the amount of active tissue. With a decrease in amount of active testes there is a decrease in content of fatty acids. For the femme fatale, fatty acids are also essential for good skin.

A recent discovery in medicine is the prostaglandins. Their full function is still not clear, but they seem to be very much involved in reproductive processes. Originally this series of substances was found in high amounts in the prostate secretion and in the semen, and their presence seemed to be essential for sperm viability and important in ejaculation. In fact, there seems to be a relationship between semen and relaxation of the female's uterus. Because the relaxation response seems to be highest in mid-cycle (around the time of ovulation), the hypothesis that the semen contains a substance that facilitates the passage of sperm by way of relaxation of the uterus seems logical. On the other hand, the pregnant uterus undergoes contraction when exposed to semen, giving credibility to tales of labor coming soon after sexual activity in pregnant women. The sedation effects of the prostaglandins have been correlated with the sleep response after sexual activity. Absence of the essential fatty acids from the diet will lead to a decreased production of prostaglandins.

In animals such as chickens, rats, and rabbits, a deficiency of essential fatty acids results in decreased reproductive ability.

The liver and pancreas have the most to do with the breakdown and absorption of fats in man. This can offer a partial explanation for decreased sexual functioning in people with diseases of these glands.

The essential fatty acids are found in ample quantity in oils derived from plants, such as corn oil, olive oil, and safflower oil. Fatty acids for femmes fatales and prostaglandins for the potent depend on maintenance of adequate fat in the diet, particularly fats from plants—meat fats tend to contain more cholesterol and less in the way of essential fatty acids.

Ambergris

From the sperm whale, ambergris is now used mostly in perfumery. Up to the nineteenth century it was used as flavoring in syrups and sauces, and was reported to have aphrodisiac qualities. Since it contains steroidlike substances this claim might have had a basis in fact. Now it is out of fashion and very expensive. It was just about unobtainable even in the nineteenth century, though Brillat-Savarin recommended adding it to chocolate as a restorative after nights of excess.

Tobacco

Tobacco is one thing, a cigarette another. Heavy cigarette smoking involves more than just nicotine—it leads to the accumulation of large amounts of carbon monoxide in the blood, which impairs an efficient supply of oxygen to the cells. Thus, heavy smoking tends to decrease sexual capabilities. Nicotine, on the other hand, can act as a glandular stimulant and in small amounts can stimulate sexuality. For those tobacco lovers who want to avoid the poisons in the smoke, chewing tobacco is the best alternative (providing your sex partner is understanding).

Trace Metals for Men

Zinc

A man needs zinc for erections. Just a few years ago the trace elements were barely measurable. However, zinc deficenc has been traced to loss of sexual potency in men.

With each ejaculation, zinc is lost. As sexual activity becomes more vigorous there must be zinc replacement to keep balance.

To start earlier in the zinc story, the question must be raised as to what happens if zinc is continuously deficient. In 1966, Dr. A. S. Prasad and his colleagues published a book about zinc and man (Charles C. Thomas, 1966). In it he described some dwarfs who had infantile sex organs even at the age of 21 whose condition could be corrected with a supplement of 100 milligrams of zinc sulfate daily. One of the reasons for the deficiency was a substance called phytate, found in unleavened bread and other food sources, which attached itself to dietary zinc and prevented it from being absorbed into the body.

Food processing removes a great deal of zinc from food. For example, approximately 80 percent of the zinc in wheat flour is removed in the milling process. In the past, some bread companies have expressed pleasure at the elimination of so much zinc—it allows the bread to keep longer because bugs won't grow on it. But the bugs aren't so dumb either—they need the zinc and get it from other sources.

Foods prepared in copper cookware also may cause a zinc problem since the copper antagonizes the zinc in the body. Zinc is also found in the liquid surrounding canned foods which often is just thrown down the drain.

Once again the lowly oyster comes through in a sexual pinch—there are approximately 120 milligrams of zinc in one-fourth of a pound of oysters.

Zinc is associated closely with histamine (from the amino acid histidine), and histamine has been associated with sexual behavior. One study indicates that women who do not achieve orgasm have low histamine levels (and lower zinc levels since the two seem to travel together). Keeping histidine at a good level may be important. Folic acid therapy will increase the level of histamine in the tissues. Much of the research about zinc and histamine in sexual behavior has not been fully documented; there is enough evidence to warrant its mention—but not its endorsement.

Dr. Carl Pfeiffer of the Brain Bio Institute in Princeton, New Jersey, is a strong advocate of the importance of zinc. He feels that a zinc-deficient girl may have delayed onset of menstruation or menstrual difficulties. He uses zinc and vitamin B_6 for these cases and claims success. He also prescribes zinc supplements for impotent men, but indicates that the therapy may take six months. This illustrates one of the problems in evaluating a claim regarding zinc therapy. Over a six-month period there can be tremendous changes in life, removal of particular stresses, and normal curing and healing. This might also be six months of psychotherapy. Can we rightfully give credit to the zinc?

Foods rich in zinc include oysters and herring. Meats are good sources. Fruits and nuts have relatively little. Pure wheat bran is a good cereal source but by weight only one-tenth as good as Casanova's oyster.

Cadmium

This is mentioned only to note that it antagonizes the action of zinc in the body. The amount of metal that goes into food after it has been cooked in a cadmium pot will vary. It is known that using old-fashioned copper cookware often results in a high copper level in food, so cookware should be considered. Cadmium is also found in cigarette smoke, in water where the household plumbing is old and in water and food contaminated by industrial wastes.

Magnesium

This is needed for proper sexual functioning and like zinc it is lost through ejaculation. Magnesium deficiency is relatively frequent in alcoholics. Perhaps this goes along with the reduced libido common in heavy drinkers.

Spermine and Spermidine

These are the twins that give human semen its characteristic odor. A good protein source is needed to keep these amines coming along the body's synthesis pathways.

The Fly Agaric

Previously some mention was made of the magic mushroom, *Psilocybe cubensis,* which has not been known as a particular sex stimulant. In fact, the opposite is true—it has figured more in nonphysically oriented spiritual and religious ceremonies.

The fly agaric (*Amanita muscaria*) is a different story indeed. This mushroom, crowned by a golden orange, red, or crimson and speckled top, figured prominently in fertility rites and sexual initiations.

Even the manner in which the mushroom was ingested and then reingested points toward some sexual functions. In Siberia, tribal elders generally ate the mushroom first. Then, because the active substance is excreted unchanged in the urine, the elders' urine was drunk by the next senior tribe members, and so on. Finally the urine was disposed of, and cavorting reindeer, attracted by the salt in the urine, have been described.

These rites were closely associated with harvest rituals and rituals to influence the quantity and quality of offspring. The effects upon sexual urges are seen more clearly in accounts of the Middle Ages where the fly agaric was used by witches and reports of wild and crazed orgies were common.

Vegetarianism

Strict vegetarianism tends to result in a decreased sexual urge and capability unless care is taken to provide supplements. First, protein is essential, and a varied source of proteins is needed. For example, while it is true that the soybean is an excellent source of protein, it also contains thyroid-inhibiting properties—and an active thyroid is essential for sexuality. Therefore, nuts, beans, whole cereals, and other sources should be mixed.

Another protein consideration involves the varying proportions of amino acids in different plants. Tryptophan, an important amino acid, is in extremely low concentration in corn. Cereals are short in the amino acid lysine while soybeans are low in methionine. Thus the strict vegetarian must plan a well-balanced protein diet for sexual functioning, whereas the meat/animal products eater and the vegetarian who eats milk and eggs do not need to be as concerned about balance.

Vitamin B_{12} is found almost exclusively in meats and animal products, and a mild deficiency state can result. However, because folic acid is plentiful in green vegetables, the symptoms of anemia characteristic of vitamin B_{12} deficiency will be masked.

Meat is a good source of zinc, but also many vegetables contain phytic acids and phytates which bind calcium, zinc, and other trace metals, preventing them from being absorbed. Foods with this binding ability include beans, other legumes, and grains.

Ferments with a Fizz

Alcohol in excess is a real sexual spoiler for men. Alcohol is a funny food-drug in that the dosage ranges for "slightly high," "intoxicated," and "dead drunk" are so close.

If alcohol were a drug that was just introduced to the Food and Drug Administration it is extremely unlikely it could pass any rigorous evaluation. For example, it is desirable for a medicine to have a low therapeutic-to-toxic ratio. If the prescribed dose is one pill and a lethal dose is one hundred pills there is a ratio of 1:100. If the dose is one capsule and the toxic or lethal dose is ten capsules, then the ratio is 1:10. With alcohol, the difference between effective range and toxic or lethal range is small. Three martinis in an hour might cause impairment but be relatively safe; ten might be lethal. A ratio of 1:3 is unacceptable for any usual medication!

What this means to sexuality is that in small doses, alcohol stimulates desire and probably has little effect on male capability. In just slightly larger doses, the effect on desire might still be there but performance is impaired. At just a slightly higher level, desire is reduced and capability is nowhere. Many men with a tendency toward problems in sustaining erections find that just a small amount of alcohol brings out their difficulty.

Sexuality in women seems to be more complex than in men. Provided the setting is right and the woman is reasonably pleased with her sexual partner, small amounts of alcohol accentuate sexuality in women, probably by reducing inhibitions. In a survey of one hundred women who were asked about foods and their effects, seven volunteered the information that alcohol made them feel more sensual. None reported that it decreased their sexual urge. Subsequently, when twenty young women were specifically asked about this, twelve reported that alcohol made them feel more sensual.

Spanish Fly—A Crash Landing

No discussion of foods and sex can be complete without a mention of Spanish fly, or cantharides. How it got its reputation as an aphrodisiac is hidden, and for good reason. The major property of Spanish fly is that it produces striking irritation of the bladder and the urethra (the small tube that brings urine out from the bladder). It is such an irritant that even death has been reported from its use. And there is no evidence that it stimulates sexuality at all. With all the pain produced, however, it probably mimics the irritation that might come from twenty-four hours of nonstop sexual activity.

The active substance to be avoided is contained in the beetle (not a fly at all). When enough of the beetles are dried up and pulverized a high level of active cantharidin results. Of some interest is that a very dilute solution has been said to stimulate hair growth, and it is still in use for that purpose, although definite results have not been demonstrated. The irritation and increased blood supply to the area have been the basis for such treatment.

9 Foods for Talking

There are some foods that can be expected to induce and stimulate the flow of talk at any get-together.

While there are many other means of communication between people, talk remains the most frequently employed and is often a source of great pleasure. People get off on talk and when there is good, satisfying conversation, they have a sense of well-being. As psychologists and psychiatrists of our day have discovered, talk itself can have cathartic effects.

But often when people come together in unfamiliar surroundings with people they do not know well, they feel inhibited and there is a dearth of talk. The silence weighs heavily, and nothing makes a host or hostess feel worse than seeing his or her guests mute. The central nervous system basis for such inhibition probably relates to some ancient survival advantage—a state of vigilance among strangers—which no longer is as relevant today. In *Beyond the Pleasure Principle*, Freud wrote of a "protective shield" of the more advanced areas of the brain that serves to limit extraneous stimuli. Such a shield or state of vigilance is a barrier to relaxation and social interaction.

The chemical action of foods can help stimulate talk as well as provide the comfort that comes from "breaking bread." There are two major types of foods that stimulate talk—slight depressants which dull inhibitions (e.g., alcohol); and stimulants (e.g., coffee). If we think of the "shield" as being an outer shell, the shell can be weakened by diminishing it or by overriding it from inside.

Start with cheese. Aged cheese contains tyramine, a central nervous system stimulant with properties similar to those of amphetamine (known to produce garrulous and even nonstop talking) and cocaine. Aged Cheddar, Brie, bleu cheese, and Stilton are all good choices. Avoid processed cheese spreads since they may not be aged at all.

Pickled herring is another good choice, and chicken livers, while less effective, share this talk-inducing property. The effect can be found with any food that has the amino acid tyrosine which changes to tyramine during aging, fermentation, pickling, etc.

Wine has long been known to relax people. Most red wines have greater tranquilizing effects than white wines (see chapter 12 for further details on wines and their effects). With strong cheese red wines (except Chianti) tend to soften the edges produced by the nervous system stimulation. On the other hand, if aged cheese is not served, a wine with some stimulant properties of its own can be effective. Such wines as Chianti and sangria are good. Another choice is a good champagne. Beer has mixed effects.

Coca-Cola was perhaps one of the most effective social drinks. During the late 1800s and early 1900s, its combination of cocaine, alkaloids of the kola nut (predominantly caffeine), and other flavorings and sugar made it a chemically powerful mixture. A decade or two before the introduction of Coca-Cola, *vin mariani* was a much-praised mixture of wine and cocaine.

Coffee—The Talk Food of Our Time

Coffee was considered to be a gift of the gods to the Arabs and the Persians. There are as many different tales about its discovery as there are types of coffees.

One tale is that it was found by an Abyssinian goatherd named Kaldi who noticed his flock was friskier after eating the fruit of a glossy green tree. He tried some and felt a rush of energy. A passing monk saw him cavorting with his flock, asked the reason, and then brought some beans back to his monastery where they were used by the monks in order to stay awake all night to say prayers.

A Christian story says that the Archangel Gabriel brought the fruit to earth. A Sufi legend has it that a banished dervish named Omar was weak from exhaustion, found the coffee bean, and took it, at which time his energy returned. Bringing this miracle food back to his people he was once again accepted.

Regardless, it is clear that once coffee was introduced it caught on rapidly. By the sixteenth and seventeenth centuries many coffeehouses for meetings and camaraderie had been established. In Colonial America, the first coffeehouse was opened about 1670 in Boston by one Dorothy Jones, who applied for a license to sell "coffee and Chuchaletto." It rapidly became a household staple in the seventeenth century in Turkey, where a wife could gain a divorce on the grounds that she was denied her fair share of the coffee.

The French historian Michelet said in 1789 that the French Revolution could be traced in part to the changes in people's habits and temperaments owing to widespread drinking of coffee. Of further historical interest is that coffee drinking increased after the celebrated dumping of tea in the Boston harbor in 1773. Coffeehouses became the meeting places where the American Revolution was plotted. Growing temperance pressures directed attention toward coffee, and more than one hundred years later prohibition gave coffee a powerful push into prominence.

Like every other drug or food with a strong effect the history of coffee includes its being banned initially. Even in Mecca it was banned for a time in the sixteenth century, but the sultan liked the beverage and reinstated it. In the seventeenth century the Church tried to ban coffee, but the Pope, the final arbiter, was a coffee drinker. Soon after, cappuccino was invented as a "remedy" against plague.

Through all the controversies, coffee power has been recognized. In 1825, Brillat-Savarin crystallized this recognition when he said, "Coffee is a more powerful liquor than commonly believed. A man of sound constitution may drink two bottles of wine per day, and live long; the same man would not so long sustain a like quantity of coffee; he would become imbecile or die of consumption."

Now coffee is the most popular beverage in the world. There is active trading of over six billion pounds of it yearly.

As with every plant growing from different seeds in differing climatic conditions, there is a multiplicity of coffees containing varying amounts of caffeine and other alkaloids. For example, Brazilian coffee usually has a higher caffeine content than Colombian or Central American coffee. Coffee tasters use words that express composition differences such as "body" (thickness), "aroma" (amount and type of volatile chemicals), and "acidity" (measured by sharpness of bitterness or sourness of taste).

While chocolate has gained a reputation as a sexual stimulator and tea is promoted as a drink to aid contemplation, coffee seems to be primarily involved with social gatherings where talk and communication is much valued. However, temperance organizations sometimes campaigned against coffee as well as alcohol—and included statements about its aphrodisiac qualities in their literature.

Kola Nuts and Other Talk Stimulators

In areas where the kola nut is found, partygoers can have a treat. In addition to a stimulating flavor, the kola nut (when eaten, chewed, or made into a beverage) contains caffeine (as in coffee), theobromine (as in chocolate), kolanin (with possible stimulating effects as well), and glucose (the simplest sugar for ready use by the body).

Another beverage with a high caffeine content (usually three times that of coffee) is guarana, made from the seeds and roots of a plant native to the Amazon valley.

If the *Catha edulis* plant is to be found (it is very common in Yemen), some party stimulation will be added. Khat is called "the cocaine of Africa." The main reason it is not exported is that the leaves lose potency within twenty-four hours of being picked. Coca-Cola is a favorite accompaniment as groups of Yemenite men chew khat and cluster for their social life between midday and midnight. Women generally are not included, and while a majority of men in Yemen use khat, few women do—at least in public.

For those plant gatherers or devotees of herb stores, ephedra tea will also set the talk going. Its ephedrine content gives it antiasthma properties as well as stimulating effects.

Keeping Guests Loose with Herbs and Spices

Herbs and spices have long been known to enliven both food and conversation. They exert effects primarily by delighting the palate and the sense of smell—but that's not all. A little valerian is a good calmer and relaxant, but too much will put your guests to sleep. Saffron has been used to enliven parties and stimulate guests for hundreds of years. Sweet basil also helps to put people at ease.

Peppermint is a stimulant that has also been recognized for centuries. While its effects are usually mild, there have been reports of people who were enraptured by peppermint and ate such huge quantities that a state of excitation and toxic psychosis resulted. The active substance is menthol, which makes up half of peppermint oil. Menthol is also found in cocoa and yarrow, but in much smaller amounts. Mentholated cigarettes can also produce a slight menthol reaction.

Nutmeg and pepper can serve to enliven guests. Another stimulant is salep, which is used to replace morning coffee in the East and contains some caffeinelike substances.

With all these talk stimulants at a get-together, it is obvious what guests will talk about as they become comfortable and chatty—they will talk about all the talk foods.

If people are stimulated to talk and socialize, they interact—and interaction leads to action. Foods that stimulate talk have probably had more influence upon civilization than any others. When Alexander Pope talked about "Coffee which makes the politicians wise," he was recognizing the effects of stimulating speech. Richelieu noted that "The government of a nation is often decided over a cup of coffee."

10 Foods and Learning

Homo sapiens is a very unusual creature. Take a large mammal, like a horse. A colt is born and within a half-hour, it can walk. While still relying on its mother for feeding, it can be relatively independent after a month. But a human is literally helpless for months and years, and the growth of the brain and learning and intelligence is a marvel.

There are ten billion nerve cells in the brain, all little energy generators, and the number of connections between the cells staggers the imagination. When people "put their minds to it," we get great achievements—the pyramids, airplanes, computers. The great neurophysiologist Sir Charles Sherrington is reported to have said, "The complexity of the brain staggers even its own imagination."

In order to develop, the brain requires millions of complex chemical interactions, but at the base of them all is good nutrition. Millions of years of food gathering has shown mankind which foods are edible. The knowledge those years has provided is now being challenged by the food industry, which removes natural substances and adds chemical foolers. The tremendous number of chemical additives and artificial foods developed over the past twenty-five years may represent chemical interference in ways we may not now even guess. The arrogance of tampering for purposes of more lively color (who cares if the pickle is light green or dark green?) and commercial success is colossal. Long-term effects on our brain must await, in most cases, a critical evaluation of history—it takes years to detect trends. If the deficiencies are subtle, they may go totally undetected.

The brain has myriad patterns of electrical energy running through it. Sherrington philosophically described it as "an enchanted loom where millions of flashing shuttles weave a dissolving pattern, always a meaningful pattern, though never an abiding one." Much of the function of the brain is still unknown, and the nature of consciousness rests in realms of philosophy.

However, we do know some important things. For one, we know that what we call memory or learning is associated with the formation of new proteins in specific areas. Ribonucleic acid (RNA) is associated with memory storage and learning. It is the chemical substance in the nerve cell that acts as a messenger telling the cell what and how much new protein to make. The cell functions as though it were a factory where the boss gives the orders to the lieutenants, who go off to tell the workers what machinery to adjust. The RNA is the lieutenant of the cell. Substances that either block protein synthesis or inactivate or block the RNA cause learning impairment.

Studies on the planaria show that when one of these small organisms eats a fellow planaria that has been trained, it either seems to learn what the other planaria had learned or its learning is facilitated in some way. This might relate to the cannibalism of Neanderthal man who ate his fellow human's brain, and might thereby have accelerated some types of learning.

The key to learning seems to be the stimulation of new

protein synthesis. In order for this to occur there must be suitable external stimulation and a suitable response. The response involves the presence of the building blocks (from food), the transport systems to get them to the right place, the stimulation that induces learning and memory, the membranes that allow entry of ions and needed material, the cellular factory which prepares the new protein pattern, and many complex chemical-electrical interactions.

Proteins for Mental Power

While there are twenty common amino acids which make up proteins, some of them can be synthesized by the body but not always in the quantities needed. The amino acids that cannot be made are tryptophan, phenylalanine, lysine, threonine, valine, methionine, leucine, and isoleucine. Some of these are important particularly in the brain and are vital to the nervous system function.

Serotonin is made from tryptophan and seems to have a great deal to do with controlling cycles, adaptation, and spiritual states. Phenylalanine and tyrosine provide the base for synthesis of norepinephrine, an important chemical messenger having to do with drives, sexuality, and other functions including learning.

Some of the amino acids seem to act as stimulators or inhibitors of the nerve cells themselves. For example, glycine seems to be a postsynaptic inhibitor (it acts to inhibit the impulse after it has formed). Excess glycine results in lethargy.

Glutamic acid is another amino acid transmitter that is involved in nerve cell processes. It has been used therapeutically in reducing convulsions. A 1944 report by Drs. Frederick Zimmerman and Sherman Ross in the *Archives of Neurology and Psychiatry* described enhancement of maze-learning ability in white rats that were given supplements of glutamic acid. The next step was to determine if supplements would cause good effects in children. There are some reports of IQ increases of five to twenty points for many patients with mild or moderate mental retardation. However, not all studies have confirmed this.

Protein supplementation might initially seem to be a good idea, but a difficulty can arise from imbalances of amino acids. Excess leucine can result in low blood sugar in some people. When children were given extra methionine some developed decreased appetite and lesser ability to retain any protein. Excess glutamate has caused symptoms of discomfort like the Chinese Restaurant Syndrome from too much mon-osodium glutamate. The best alternative to supplementation is to use protein-rich foods that are naturally balanced. The effects of single amino acid supplements emphasize that an amino acid is or can be thought of as a drug.

The Cactus and Concentration

When people speak of learning they do not usually separate it into types. But there are two large subdivisions of learning—positive learning and negative learning. Positive learning is learning something because it is useful in life, gives happiness in some way, or is interesting. Negative learning is learning what not to do.

Parents teach a child in many ways, but at opposite poles are teaching by example and teaching solely by punishment. The first is the most positive way and the second is the most negative. Eating peyote cactus reduces the retention of material learned by the negative means, but does not affect positive learning. This is similar to the effect of low doses of LSD on learning, and the same holds true for the psilocybin mushroom.

Alcohol, except perhaps at very low doses, reduces all

forms of learning. This is probably a result of an overall inhibition or slowing of protein synthesis. In addition, alcohol has a direct effect on proteins and actually causes characteristic changes in some amino acids. All substances tested that reduce protein synthesis also reduce learning. But alcohol may have even more of a negative effect because of its alteration effects which result in increases of GABA, an inhibiting substance in the brain. This may well be a possible reason for alcoholism. That is, feel bad, drink and feel better, get more inhibition, feel even worse, drink to feel better, and so on and so on.

Tea for Tests

There are many, many substances that slow learning, and they can come through foods. But what can help?

One that can is tea made from the ephedra plant. Ephedrine, similar to amphetamine, is widely used to treat conditions such as asthma. Perhaps by simply helping to open the air passages and allowing in more oxygen, or by some central nervous system stimulation, this tea can facilitate learning. This has been the subject of many scientific reports which confirm some beneficial effects at low doses. Some people also feel that it can enhance athletic performance. In fact, it was ephedrine that a swimmer said he had been taking for his asthma, which led to his disqualification in the Olympic Games at Mexico City in 1968.

Ephedra tea also has a mild aphrodisiac effect, and since the ephedra plant grows wild in the Nevada deserts, it has been served for many years in some mobile brothels. Its nickname is "whorehouse tea." Perhaps an added benefit was that customers could remember their experiences better.

Caffeine in coffee and theophylline in tea aid learning through cerebral stimulation. Similar effects occur from the coca plant and khat, the mint green leaf of the shrub *Catha edulis,* which is widely used in Africa and Yemen. The kola nut, also a caffeine source, will assist in learning.

Certain teas also have mental stimulant effects which can aid retention. For example, peppermint tea has menthol, a stimulant. Small amounts of pepper might be beneficial as well.

What should be avoided are depressants such as beer (which contains hops, a sedative), valerian, jasime tea, thyme, and marijuana. These will work against learning of academic material.

In our society we generally think of learning in a framework of "reading, writing, and arithmetic." But there is another sort of learning, which might involve the opposite side of the brain. This sort of artistic comprehension might be aided by some depressants. As Pliny the Elder said, *In vino veritas* ("In wine is the truth"). A. E. Housman poems extolled beer thusly:

> Oh many a peer of England brews
> Livelier liquor than the Muse,
> And malt does more than Milton can
> To justify God's ways to man.
> Ale, man, ale's the stuff to drink
> For fellows whom it hurts to think:
> Look into the pewter pot
> To see the world as the world's not.

11 ⟋ High-Powered Foods

"Don Juan spoke with deep fervor about Mescalito's being the teacher of the proper way to live," says Carlos Castañeda in *The Teachings of Don Juan*.

It is a humble plant, this *Lophophora williamsii*, a small cactus barely rising half a foot from the ground and growing wild through parts of Mexico, Texas, Arizona, and New Mexico. Its history is shrouded with mystery as befits such a highly venerated vegetable.

The Aztecs worshiped three plants. One they called teonactl, or "flesh of the gods," another was ololiuqui, and the third was peyotl, the unassuming cactus. This last vegetable produced such strange alterations in the usual perception of reality that the Indians felt that a god, Mescalito, resided within it. This god provided grain and maize for the body and peyote for the spirit.

The sacred cactus is gathered in October, just before the dry season in Mexico. For the Indians even the gathering is a religious experience. The fleshy top, or button, is cut into sections, allowed to dry, and becomes like a small wrinkled plant covered with thin whitish hairs. The active ingredient is mescaline, which physicians call a hallucinogen.

Many Americans have tried this vegetable, some finding its effects profound and meaningful. Aldous Huxley's *Doors of Perception,* written in 1954, is primarily about the new insights and view of the world he achieved with it. For many, taking peyote results in an orgy of visual changes. One remarkable effect is the production of colors not ordinarily seen.

Whether these perceptions represent toxic effects or an expansion of consciousness is still not established. While the debate was at its peak, in the 1950s, its use in the United States was declared illegal except by the Native American Church of North America as part of their ritual. Legal cacti with similar effects are the donaña cactus and the San Pedro cactus—but the extraction process is more difficult.

The potent effect on the mind produced by the sacred cactus points out a major theme of this book: Foods contain chemical substances that exert effects on people. Most of the foods we eat exert subtle effects because the concentrations of the active substances are low.

Peyote and Healing

Indian shamans have used the peyote for healing. Its effects don't seem to be specific, but perhaps it allows insights to reduce mental conflict and so reduces mental illnesses that can arise from such conflict—depressions, for example. With the reduction of psychic tension, diseases that seem to arise from imbalances within the nervous system—so-called psychosomatic illnesses—may be reduced. Also, the awakening of religion often seen might allow for the relaxation that can come from a mystical experience and prayer. The effects of mescaline on hormones and the immune system of the body have barely been studied. Indians who take peyote frequently are—despite poverty, sometimes inadequate nutrition, and insufficient doctors—healthy and long-lived. Of possible importance is the ability of mescaline to reduce pain.

Seeking the Eternal Magic Mushroom

Not content with supermarket mushrooms, during the early spring and summer, mushroom lovers may be found scouring the fields and cow pastures for the *Psilocybe cubensis.* They are seeking the strange experiences that result from the voyages of the mind effected by this mushroom, found throughout the southern United States and in the West, particularly in Oregon and Washington. Those with limited knowledge should stay away from the mushroom fields because there are varieties of mushrooms with toxic chemicals that cause severe nausea, vomiting, abdominal pain, and diarrhea. Some can cause liver damage or damage to the brain and kidneys; some can be fatal.

It is widely believed that mushrooms are edible, poisonous, or "magic"—that is, containing the psychoactive substance called psilocybin. In fact, even some "edible" types may contain very small amounts of psychoactive substances, while some of the "poisonous" varieties have been used— cautiously—for their mind-changing effects.

The mushroom is actually the fruit of a fungus. People have pointed out that what we don't eat is a network of filaments underneath the ground extending as much as one hundred feet into topsoil. This network is symbolic of the varied interconnections of the physical and spiritual world which we do not even begin to realize. As with all such plants of power, a religious cult grew around magic mushrooms, and experiencing these mushrooms seems to bring man and religion much closer.

The history of mushrooms and psychic power are intimately intertwined with stories of "fairy food" and elves.

Lewis Carroll's *Alice in Wonderland* may have resulted from
the author's experience with mushrooms. Dr. Albert Hoffman, famed biochemist and discoverer of LSD, also synthesized psilocybin, the main psychedelic substance of the magic
mushroom. He tested the mushrooms first on himself and
was so intrigued that he continued work on the strange
substance.

Gordon Wasson, once a banker, became so interested
in the psilocybin mushroom after trying it that he left his
work and became the world's leading mushroom expert. He
has speculated that the origins of religion may be traced to
uses of the mushroom, and feels that perhaps the apple of
the Bible which opened men's and women's eyes to good
and evil was actually a mushroom. The Aztecs named the
psilocybin mushroom "teonactl" because they believed that
a god resided in it.

While we are used to foods with little power of altering
consciousness, effects may be seen even from one mushroom,
although usually six or twelve are taken. Chocolate seems to
heighten the effects. One interesting finding by Robert
Graves, the poet and mystic, is that the initials of the Greek
words for ambrosia ("nectar of the gods") spell the Greek
word for mushroom. Graves has further speculated that the
feasts of Dionysus were really mushroom orgies rather than
drinking feasts. He also suggests that the divine food soma,
written about in the Hindu Rig-Veda, was actually a hallucinogenic strain of mushroom.

But what about other mushrooms often termed poisonous? A principal example is the *Amanita muscaria,* the fly
agaric found throughout Europe, Asia, and North America,
which frequently grows at the base of trees. This mushroom
looks just like the typical toadstool which has been a favorite
motif in art and children's books. There is some interesting
historical information about this mushroom which sheds
some light on its effects.

When fly agaric is eaten in moderate quantities, its main active ingredient, muscarine, produces a kind of rage reaction. The Vikings were said to use it prior to going into battle, and there are tales of superhuman feats of strength resulting from its use. Because of the association between muscarine and acetylcholine, ordinarily responsible for muscular action, there is a basis for such stories. The strange effects of this mushroom also led to its use by witches through the ages.

Another active substance in the fly agaric is ibotenic acid which causes changes in sensory perceptions. Overdosage of this mushroom is highly dangerous. Other mushrooms of the genus *Amanita* also can contain toxins made of amino acids in complex chemical configurations. They are highly toxic to man, so neophyte mushroom hunters must learn to identify them.

Nutmeg—The Holiday Favorite

The dried seed of the plant *Myristica fragrans* is the easily obtainable nutmeg. Its active ingredients apparently are myristin (also in black pepper and dill), safrole, and pinene. The effects of nutmeg include distortion of time and place, feelings of unreality, and, occasionally, marked visual hallucinations. The search for nutmeg and pepper in the fifteenth, sixteenth, and seventeenth centuries bears witness to the high value placed upon these psychoactive spices; Spanish galleons were sent out with gold to trade for pepper.

Dr. Robert Schulze (July 15, 1976) reported in the prestigious *New England Journal of Medicine* that when he served as medical officer in a Caribbean prison he noticed that nutmeg was frequently enclosed in food parcels sent to inmates. The nutmeg was eaten, sniffed, or smoked with tobacco.

Other Hallucinogenic Plants

It is remarkable how many mind-altering plants there are around the world and how they have been discovered and used by natives in the area. There are at least forty known hallucinogenic vegetables.

Species of *Piptadenia* and *Mimosa* produce a substance that South American Indians have found will produce hallucinations when eaten or used as snuff. The active compound is similar to mescaline. The Waika Indians in South America use epena, which comes from a nutmeglike tree. Natives of Brazil, Colombia, and Peru use a beverage called caapi or ayahuasca from plants of the genus *Banisteria* to produce dreams that foretell the future. Also in South America we find the yage, which has a hallucinogenic effect like that of LSD. The tribal medicine man prepares the yage drink; a translation of his chant, from Andrew Weil's *The Natural Mind*, gives some idea of what is expected:

> Vision Vine
> Boding spirit of the forest
> origin of our understanding
> give up your magic power
> to our potion
> illuminate our mind
> bring us foresight
> show us the design of our enemies
> expand our knowledge
> expand our understanding
> of our forest.

The seeds of *Peganum harmala*, which have been used as a spice, contain harmine, otherwise called telepathine because of its psychic effects. Not only will this plant induce hallucinations, but its active substance is similar to a hormone of the pineal gland.

Natives of certain sections of Africa chew the root of a

shrublike plant called *Tabernanthe iboga,* with excitement and hallucinations occurring shortly after.

In Mexico, one of the three plants worshiped by the Aztecs was ololiuqui (*Rivea corymbosa*). The seeds from this plant have LSD-like effects. Closer to home, it appears that the same substances are found in the seeds of the morning glory (*Ipomoea violacea*). Hawaiian baby wood rose seeds have similar effects.

The seeds and leaves of the common jimson weed can produce hallucinations owing to their alkaloid content. Similar effects can come from eating the leaves of tomato or potato plants. And, of course, in this day and age we cannot overlook the vegetable marijuana which is eaten, smoked, and used as seasoning.

Because of U.S. laws against substances like marijuana, searches to find alternatives have led to the discovery and importation of a wide variety of psychoactive plants. One such is the kavakava (*Piper methysticum*) of Hawaii, a plant of the pepper family. In Fiji, it is prepared by young men and women who chew the roots and spit them into a large pot; the mixture is then heated and served as a tea. Apparently the chewing helps to release the active substance, a compound called kawine. When a cup of the tea is taken, a feeling of mild intoxication and well-being results.

Foods of the Witches

"Because ye have said 'We have made a covenant with death, and with hell are we at agreement . . .' " is found in Isaiah (28:15).

While mentioned in the Bible, the concept of witchcraft or the "black arts" really took shape in the Middle Ages as the Church assumed more power. The view of life as an unceasing battle between the powers of heaven and the powers of hell was accepted and the faithful were vigilant, ready to detect any trace of Satan or his disciples. Those who made a pact with the devil were supposedly imbued with powers to cast spells on their neighbors that rendered them ill or caused their cattle and family to die. Disease was so rampant that a person who wished another ill could live to see it happen often enough to perpetrate the idea of the power of the devil.

As in the 1950s in America when those called pinkos were persecuted, in the Middle Ages the label of "witch" was often applied to political enemies. Joan of Arc was burned at the stake in 1431 after being declared a witch. The Jews, a scapegoat throughout history, were often accused of witchcraft. When children were born with congenital malformations, the mother was automatically thought to be a witch. The penalty was death, stemming from the biblical admonition "Thou shalt not suffer a witch to live" (Exodus 22:18). The presence of witches doing evil was so accepted that in the eleventh century several books were written that actually divide witches into many batallions of the devil, each with unique identifying marks.

There were men and women who considered themselves witches and met in groups (covens). Many became experts in the chemical powers of herbs. In fact, a claim could be made that clinical pharmacology owes a great debt to witches and poisoners throughout history. Witches' brews were composed of a wide variety of plants, animal parts, herbs, and spices, and were prepared for specific purposes. Early in the history of witchcraft, witches' feasts were often held with those present performing the Christian sacraments in reverse. The potions ingested for these rituals were not the poisons, which were for enemies, but included many substances that could induce hallucinations and altered states of consciousness. The brews contained ingredients such as the following.

Toad Skin

Found as part of many witches' brews was the skin of a toad. Chemical analysis reveals that it contains a substance called bufotenine, which is hallucinogenic at a very low dosage, with effects similar to those of LSD.

Toadstools

Some toadstools also contain bufotenine. Mushrooms of the genus *Psilocybe* induce tremendous sensory distortions and hallucinations because they contain psilocybin. Other mushrooms, such as *Amanita muscarina,* have a potent substance that stimulates a portion of the nervous system. Excess amounts can produce tremendous glandular secretion, frothing at the mouth, and visual hallucinations.

Meadow Saffron

Also called autumn crocus and wild saffron, this was a frequent component of witches' brews. It contains colchicine, an important medicine used to treat gout. In excess this drug causes severe abdominal pain, nausea, vomiting, diarrhea, burning of the mouth and throat, and, in larger dosages, muscular paralysis and death from asphyxiation. In small amounts colchicine has anti-inflammatory actions and gives some people a sense of well-being. Meadow saffron is different from the saffron used for seasoning.

Deadly Nightshade

Also added to witches' brews, this plant appears in Greek history. The major active ingredient is atropine, one of the belladonna alkaloids, a potent medication that inhibits many glandular functions, causes dilation of the eyes, and in larger dosages causes confusion and hallucinations. Death can result from extremely large dosages. The potato is a member of this plant family, and when the leaves of the potato plant are eaten a similar syndrome results. The same holds true for the eggplant. Some of the juices from this plant have been used by women—Cleopatra, for example—who put it into their eyes for the dilating effects; hence the name belladonna ("beautiful lady").

The devil's weed, or nightshade, was one of the plants the Yaqui Indian witch doctor gave to Carlos Castañeda, who wrote about his experiences in *The Teachings of Don Juan.* Like the witches of old, Castañeda anointed his body with the crushed plant, and describes feeling as if he were flying at great speed around the mountains. The separate reality concept was explored the next day when Castañeda asked whether he had really flown, and Don Juan told him that he flew like a man who has taken the devil's weed.

Hemlock (Conium Fruit)

This witches' plant is found throughout Europe, Asia, and America. It is said to be the one used by Socrates in his suicide. In large doses it can cause weakness, drowsiness, and paralysis leading to death. Some modern poisonings have resulted from eating quail that have feasted on hemlock seed, which is practically harmless to them.

The sometimes close relationship between foods and toxic substances can be seen in another member of the same family, parsley, which is commonly eaten and is harmless in usual quantities.

Wolfsbane (Monkshood)

This plant has been used in medicine in very low dosages, but from early Greek history it was used in witches' potions. Containing aconitine, it is toxic to the heart.

Verbena

This is a component of Greek witches' potions, and comes from the plant *Verbena officinalis* which causes nausea and vomiting. In large doses it depresses the heart and makes the heartbeat irregular.

Poppies

Poppies are used for their opium and other alkaloids from which we get the very useful morphine and the not so useful heroin. These alkaloids acted as a sedative and euphoriant in witches' brews, but in large dosages caused death.

Henbane

This was part of brews from the Middle Ages on, and was said to conjure demons. Because of its content of scopolamine, a very potent drug, it can cause flushing, dilated pupils, and confusion with bizarre hallucinations. The mouth becomes dry and the glands are inhibited. During the Korean War, scopolamine was used for brainwashing, and because it caused loss of control over speech content it was thought to be a truth serum. It used to be popular in obstetrics to induce twilight sleep, but side effects were frequent.

Laurel

Laurel contains morphinelike substances in its leaves and bark. In ancient Greece use of the laurel was associated with an altered state of consciousness and was believed to aid in prophecy. Apollo's prophetess ate and smoked it. (Cedar smoke was also felt to invoke divine powers—certainly it does produce a trance and, in some cases, convulsions.)

Mandrake

This plant has a varied history. When a man is hanged, the effect on the spinal cord may cause an ejaculation right before death. The mandrake was said to arise from the ejaculate of those who died from hanging. It was a part of witches' brews because of its irritation to the skin and the severe diarrhea it caused when eaten.

Miscellaneous Components

Often the most bizarre and gruesome substances were put into the witches' brew. These did not seem to have much effect chemically, but certainly emotionally they were potent fear inducers. Part of a dead child dug up after decaying, or even an entire dead child was cooked. Other macabre ingredients were used, including rancid food and blood from animals. Heavy metals such as copper, arsenic, lead, and mercury were used for poisonings. Modern polluters put similar poisons into our waterways.

12 Spirits, Alcohols, Wines, Other Ferments

Throughout history people have enjoyed drinking their fermented brews. Who first developed ferments? Nobody had to. Nature provided yeast which could act on sugar-containing substances to form alcohol and, in the course of the fermentation process, hundreds of other chemical compounds.

Wines

Wine has been described as a "chemical symphony" containing various alcohols, at least half a dozen vitamins, fifteen to twenty minerals, and more than twenty organic acids. There are also proteins and amino acids in it. The major components of the bouquet result from compounds called esters. Older wines may contain more than thirty-five different esters, each adding a different element to the smell. Then there are the pigments—particularly in red wines, but also in rosés and in very small amounts in white wines. Pigments also change with age and there might be fifty or one hundred forms in one wine. Wine lovers who cultivate their taste sensations can detect a variety of the compounds, which adds to their enjoyment.

Wine making depends on many variables, including type of grape, soil, amount of sunlight, temperature, time of harvest, and technique—all these before fermentation and aging have even started.

Wine power has been recognized from earliest writings and has found a secure place in mythology through Dionysus, or Bacchus (the god of wine). His name has become synonymous with the wild and drunken frenzy of parties. In mythology Dionysus was also associated with agriculture, and according to one legend pomegranates sprang from his blood.

The variety of effects of wine are well known. One extreme can be seen in Milton's verse: "Bacchus, that first from out the purple grape/ Crushed the sweet poison of misused wine." "Misused" is a key word, for in Proverbs (27: 15) it is said, "Give wine unto those that be of heavy heart"— a good suggested use. Shakespeare wrote, "Good wine is a good familiar creature if it be well used" (*Othello,* II, iii). However, recognizing the negative side of its use he also wrote, "I am falser than vows made in wine" (*As You Like It,* III, v).

To understand the effects, it is necessary to look specifically at some of the compounds present in wine. First let's look at the alcohol content. Most wines have about 12 percent alcohol, unlike distilled spirits which may have 50 percent alcohol. Unless a relatively large amount is taken the effects of this relatively low alcohol content involve an initial slight stimulation followed by a mild dulling. However, with the fortified wines, such as port with a 20 percent alcohol content, there is much more of a dulling effect. Thus fortified wines are usually better sleep inducers or calmers.

Another compound is the chemical GABA (gamma hydroxybutyric acid) which deserves mention because it is an inhibitory chemical transmitter in the brain, and has been associated with the sleep mechanism. Wines with more of it are likely to be better sleep inducers. For example, Burgundy has more than Bordeaux, which provides one explanation for a greater calming effect of the Burgundies. Sherry also is relatively high in GABA, and with its higher alcohol content it is a good before-bed wine.

Certain wines such as champagne undergo refermentation after the initial fermentation process. In France, the wine is made in late summer and initial fermentation takes place. As winter arrives or there is a particularly cold October or November, the yeast cells become inactive prior to complete fermentation. This means that there is still sugar present and cold-inactivated yeast. When the warm days come again in the spring, the yeast cells are reactivated and fermentation continues. Since the bottles are corked after the first fermentation, the second fermentation results in the production of carbon dioxide which has no way to escape, and as the pressure builds up, a sparkling wine is produced. It is possible to pump carbon dioxide into wines to imitate natural fermentation. Some sugar is added after the second fermentation process to give the champagne its required sweetness. If no more than .5 percent of sugar is added, it remains dry and is labeled *brut*. During the second fermentation process additional compounds are formed, including tyramine. The tyramine effects (stimulation and talkativeness) are part of the champagne experience, and are a possible reason that champagne is used in celebrations and has the reputation of being a truth serum.

The most famous Italian wine, widely known for its jolly qualities, is Chianti. This too undergoes a secondary fermentation and, although the gas is allowed to escape, tyramine effects are present.

The Chablis wines are said to go well with oysters. In some places Chablis has been nicknamed "oyster water." Samuel Pepys, the indefatigable diarist, reported that he always kept Chablis in his cellar specifically for drinking with oysters. This association probably resulted because Chablis grapes are grown in a chalky soil containing time-ground oyster shells—the Chablis region was underwater perhaps a million years before. The grapes and the wine are higher in iodine content, so can perk up a sluggish thyroid gland when taken frequently. The slight aphrodisiac effect of oysters and the maintenance of the thyroid gland by both the wine and the oysters can make a sexy combination.

An interesting but rare wine is called *vin jaune,* and comes from the area of France in the Jura Mountains. During its maturation a mold develops on it, giving it a slight cheesy, spicy flavor. This probably accounts for its effect, described as a special relaxation and glow.

Some wine is aged in cedar casks and assumes a different color resulting from contact with the wood. The cedar may exert other mild effects, since a slight trance state has been reported when cedar is smoked.

Vermouth is a wine with added herbs and spices such as cinchona, coriander, cinnamon, sage, thyme, and, most importantly, wormwood. Though present in small amounts, the wormwood adds a little absinthe, which has slightly euphoric effects. Thyme is a relaxer.

The staggering varieties of wines, the substances the grapes get from the soil, and the many breakdown products of the pigments have innumerable different effects. However, at this time there has not been sufficient chemical analysis of components, nor is there enough understanding of central nervous system influences to truly give due credit to all the effects. This sampling should only serve to whet interest.

Beer and Ale

Though wine was described first by the ancients, nobody knows which was the first brewed beverage. Mead, made from honey, seems to go back almost ten thousand years. Beer is also about that age, although the original brew should be called "ale" since the use of hops, a relaxant herb so much a part of modern beer, did not even begin until the end of the Middle Ages.

Simple ale is one of those fermented beverages that achieved rapid popularity because of its pleasing effects and because it is easy to make. Its inception required the development of agriculture and the cultivation of barley or other grains. The first ale was just the barley water remaining after cooking which was allowed to stand overnight and undergo fermentation.

Beer was the most popular beverage in ancient Egypt and its popularity has continued. Even in the American Colonies, beer was a frequent drink—although it didn't rival apple cider.

Food usages often reflect historical patterns of societal concerns. Beer usage changed as the American character developed. Coffee became more popular as a beverage partly because its effects were more fitting for the American work ethic. It is also possible that different foods may help stimulate societal movements. A French historian felt that the French Revolution was partially fostered by widespread coffee drinking.

Spirits (Distillates)

Societal concerns about beverages with higher alcohol content—the distillates—are obvious. Temperance movements have played a large historical role. With foods and beverages that have strong effects and are relatively easy to produce, the substances have traditionally won out. As Andrew Weil, director of the Harvard Botanical Museum, suggests, perhaps people have an innate and normal desire to periodically alter their consciousness. The differences in usage seem to reside in which strong food-drugs society tolerates. For example, we in the United States tolerate alcohol and cigarettes (perhaps because of commercial/economic factors) while outlawing other drugs. Our society tried to outlaw spirits during prohibition, but without success. One wholly approved way of altering consciousness is dietary change.

As serious drinkers know, various hard drinks have their own particular character, which exist apart from the alcohol content. But because the alcohol content is much higher than that of wine and beer, the alcohol effects are usually more pronounced. Because we are dealing with distillates, generally the salts, proteins, vitamins, and many other nutrients are not completely retained in the final products, but still provide characteristic tastes.

Brandy is the result of distillation of wine and cognac, and is often aged as long as twenty-five to forty years. Some wine pigments as well as different alcohol products are present. The principal effects involve alcohol content and taste, but some of the calming properties of wine and aging are present.

Many of the diverse effects of spirits are owing to the substances added to the mixed drinks. For example, drinks made with nutmeg result in an alcohol and nutmeg effect, and impart feelings of gaiety. Liberal amounts of nutmeg can result in an altered state of consciousness with a tendency toward mild hallucinations.

Absinthe used to be made from wormwood, which resulted in a euphoric experience; but wormwood has been outlawed and replaced by anise. The result now is a very slight stimulation. The Greek ouzo liqueur contains a resin with effects similar to those of wormwood extract.

Chocolate or coffee is added to many drinks, and the resultant stimulant actions of the caffeine and theobromine tend to offset some of the dulling effects of the alcohol.

Amaretto, which is flavored with apricot pits, is of some

interest. This is not so much because of any marked effect, but because the controversial drug laetrile, touted by some as a cancer cure, is also made from apricot pits. Some cyanide can arise from apricot pits, but in very low concentrations.

Drinks to which vanilla has been added get the mild stimulatory action of vanillin.

Tequila is one drink that has remained somewhat of a mystery. It seems to have more stimulatory properties than other distillates, but the reason is not clear. One aspect, however, can explain some effects. Tequila is often served in a Margarita with salt on the rim of the glass. The salt is an old tradition, but it serves a chemical function. Ordinarily, alcohol inhibits the production of ADH (antidiuretic hormone). As you might expect, inhibiting an antidiuretic results in diuresis—passing out of water via the urine. Salt tends to maintain the ADH. Recent research has demonstrated that the ADH has mild antidepressant properties, so using the salt and preventing the ADH decrease may result in a "happier" drink and less of a post-drink crash. This salt effect might also explain why some people insist on putting salt in their beer and why salted peanuts and chips are frequent accompaniments of alcoholic beverages.

When using an alcoholic beverage for a purpose such as sleep induction, wine is preferable. The major effect of spirits is that of alcohol, and there tends to be a rebound effect—increased excitability after it wears off.

It may be useful to look into the components of some liqueurs, although the findings may flabbergast you. For example, chartreuse, made by the Carthusian monks since 1605, contains one hundred thirty herbs and has a high alcohol content. The herbs provide some of its prized effects, which go beyond odor, taste, and alcohol.

13 Food Power Party and Entertaining Guide

What do people want from a party, and what needs do parties serve?

First, people want to get together. We have been called "social animals" which simply means that we enjoy and seek the company of others. Since a particularly highly developed human trait is speech, an important part of a party is usually verbal communication. However, there are many forms of nonverbal communication (gestures, closeness, sexual activity, "vibrations," etc.) which also go into social interactions.

The most important part of all communication is that it be effective. For this to occur people must feel comfortable and relax their emotional guards. Perhaps the tendency to tighten up among strangers is related to a complex protective mechanism, but a successful party must allow a loosening of such guards. Eating and drinking together, "breaking bread," is an important part of comfort. One of the effects of a common food-drug experience at a party is that people share a change of consciousness and become closer.

If the party has a specific purpose, the goal should be achieved—and this requires planning. For example, if the purpose of a party is to get acquainted with new business associates there must be a place for mingling to share ideas; talk would be very important. Loud music would work against talking and sharing ideas. On the other hand, if the party is planned to share nonverbal interactions, music might be just the thing to get people into dancing and body rhythms.

What makes food and drink mandatory for a party? Perhaps it harks back to a distant past where having another eat your food and share your bounty was a sign of peace and friendship, a condition essential for relaxation. Perhaps it also meant that in case of external danger you would have an ally present—another source of comfort. If so, these patterns are deeply imprinted upon man and they have affected his behavior to a large extent.

If this need is in fact an archetypal pattern or preconceived set of man's mind, there must be a strong survival advantage to it. A close band is certainly more able to defend itself than solitary individuals. There are advantages of a group of people joined together against external dangers, other tribes, and predators as well as against intergroup aggression. A group also allows for cooperative efforts and building—whether a physical construction or an abstract formulation. Moreover, the sharing of food means that those less fortunate in the hunt do not need to institute aggressive action against the one more fortunate.

Going one step further, at no time are we more vulnerable than when we are eating. For proper digestion and absorption of food, it is important for the sympathetic nervous system, the protector, to be at a low level of activity. The alternative to this is not only impairment of digestive abilities, but possible development of an ulcer of the stomach, intestinal disorders, constipation, and a whole host of diseases directly attributable to eating in a state of stress. Eating in comfort is a positive factor in both health maintenance and pleasurable mood tone.

Parties can instill a sense of well-being, from the initial invitation and feelings of acceptance by the host, hostess, and the group to the actual comfort derived from the party.

The host or hostess must provide the ingredients that will allow feelings of comfort so that guests will have their needs satisfied. The host or hostess will then derive the warm feeling of success which comes from the ability to gratify these needs. How best to do this depends upon a host's or hostess's ability to logically and intuitively sense what will be the right type of party. Farewell parties tend to be best when foods that aid in a communal feeling are served. Parties for getting to know each other better can best use talk foods. A party for brainstorming can be aided through use of foods for creativity. It all depends on what sort of party is desired. Advance planning, using food power, can help make it a success.

New Friends—A Case Study

A young married couple—Tom, aged 29, and Gretchen, aged 27—have recently moved to Smith-Town, a small suburban community. They have come because Tom, a lawyer, has joined three colleagues in a group venture. Gretchen, a teacher, does not know the women who are coming.

Tom doesn't know his business associates except in a professional capacity. Doug, aged 38, the senior member of this association, is divorced and will not be bringing a woman friend. The others—John, aged 30, and Rod, aged 35—have both been married for about eight years. Rod's wife Joan is 35. John's wife Ruth, 28, is a college graduate who is now busy at home with their two small children. For a time she worked as an assistant to a local state assemblyman.

Politically, Tom thinks John and his wife tend to be liberal Democrats, Rod is an independent, and Doug is a staunch Republican.

Party Analysis

Tom wants this initial gathering to be relatively formal—
that is, he wishes to bring out the rational/intellectual
consciousness. He feels that he would like to find out more
about his associates in terms of their beliefs, politics, orien-
tation toward life, and future plans. Gretchen, who has no
children, would like to socialize with the women to see if
they have interests in common, and with the men to find out
about them particularly in terms of their relationship with
her husband. She wants to discover their interests and she
wants to remember to include Doug even if the conversation
begins to focus on domestic and married life.

Planning

Since this is a "get to know each other," Gretchen wants
to avoid creating too intimate an atmosphere, as she could
with candlelight. The round table seems effective for this
sort of social interchange. She wants background music, but
some without words and relatively subdued so it doesn't
overpower the guests.

The place settings will be formal and she will use her
best dishes. To promote an atmosphere of individuality, she
plans to serve a dinner with discrete courses. With this
precise and formal approach she hopes to bring out critical-
analytical-worldly talk.

Food Considerations

Because the guests do not know each other well
Gretchen wants to have them immediately "break bread" to
put them at their ease. When they arrive she plans to offer
a tray of imported aged cheeses, light crispy crackers, and
wine. The reasons for these choices are important. The
cheeses offer variety and are a precise (cutting) type of food.
Moreover, Gretchen knows that the cheese contains tyramine, which acts as a brain stimulant.

Gretchen plans to offer either a red or white wine of good vintage. Though she is not a wine expert, she knows her red wine has aged for four years and has a tranquilizing effect that goes beyond its alcohol content and relates to its pigments. The white wine is very dry, and while it has fewer tranquilizing properties, it seems to go with the cheese and does offer stimulation to the taste buds. She deliberately has not considered Chianti, champagne, or sangria—they do not fit in with her planned mood and she knows that they also contain tyramine. With the cheese, the stimulation might induce a headache or overstimulation.

She also plans to have Coca-Cola available. She knows of its caffeine (stimulating) effect, and has heard that while the drug cocaine is no longer a part of "Coke," some other alkaloids from the coca plant might still be present to exert a slight euphoric effect.

At the table, the soup course will be first. Because this is to be a full-course dinner, Gretchen wants to start with a delicately flavored beef consommé. She will avoid using monosodium glutamate, knowing that it sometimes causes intestinal cramps and flushing, and tends to be a mild depressant—this may subtly work against lively table talk. Some parsley and sage will add some relaxant effects, and a little freshly ground pepper will have stimulant effects. She will avoid bean soup because it tends to be a depressant and she knows that most beans have an antithyroid factor.

Gretchen will bake her own dinner rolls, in various shapes for more interest. The warmth and aroma will add additional sensory effects. She will top them with poppy seeds, which may contain some opiumlike compounds if they are untreated.

Her salad will contain a variety of lettuces to add interest and for the mild effects of the relaxant lactucin. She will avoid tomatoes, since the only ones available were picked while green and artificially ripened in a gas chamber, so have little taste and much acidity. Bleu cheese dressing with its tyramine will stimulate talk. Fresh-ground pepper will add to this as well.

Doug will bring a Burgundy dinner wine to serve at room temperature. Burgundy tends to be somewhat more sedative than other wines so she makes a mental note to have coffee available right after the meal to offset it. She wants to keep the talk going.

For her main course Gretchen has chosen lamb chops. She knows that none of the guests are vegetarians, and she wants to avoid thick steaks which tend to induce a post-meal torpor. The lamb chop is smaller and more flavorful, and contains a high amount of the amino acid tyrosine which goes into the formation of adrenalin and thyroid hormone. She will use rosemary and borage as seasonings, knowing that they have been used for centuries for their antidepressant actions.

In addition to the green salad she wants another type of vegetable, and decides to sauté mushrooms in a small amount of butter and surround the lamb chops with them. She knows that while the mushrooms have little food power and will not chemically interact with the other foods, they have symbolic value. She plans to mention that mushrooms have filaments extending as far as one hundred feet underground and are thus symbolic of the complex interconnections and networks not visible to the eye.

For dessert Gretchen will treat her guests to a light, creamy chocolate mousse. There are many ways to prepare *mousse au chocolat,* but Gretchen chooses a recipe that includes egg whites, pure unsweetened chocolate, and an orange liqueur. A small amount of orange peel is also used for flavoring. Everyone loves chocolate mousse, but for Gretchen's party it is an especially good choice. The chocolate contains theobromine, a stimulant similar to caffeine, but perhaps a little less harsh. By dessert time, the initial stimulation from the cheese will have dissipated. Because chocolate stimulates by a different mechanism than the tyramine in the cheese, there will be no interference with the effects.

The dinner menu is planned to be light—Gretchen does not want her guests to have the feeling they might have after a Thanksgiving feast. The mousse, however, ends the meal on a rich note and is filling. It should be served in small, chilled cups with real, slivered chocolate on the top to add more chocolate—and its effects—to the menu.

Finally, coffee and after-dinner brandy. Gretchen chooses to make a coffee with chicory as they do in New Orleans. The chicory is said to induce a mild euphoria, although there is little information about it. By mixing it with the coffee, the total caffeine content is lowered. This is important because the chocolate is stimulatory and additional caffeine might result in excess sweating and feelings of discomfort.

In review, Gretchen will use food power well. The parsley and sage are relaxant herbs, and rosemary and borage are slight stimulants, as is the pepper. The initial cheese is stimulatory and talk inducing as is the later bleu cheese. Her poppy seed rolls are possibly a relaxing food while the Coca-Cola is a stimulant. The lettuce has relaxants while the coffee is stimulatory. The mushrooms offer a symbol and a topic for conversation. The Burgundy wine is a depressant while the chocolate mousse is stimulatory. The coffee with chicory adds a mild feeling of well-being.

The stimulant and relaxant effects are relatively balanced. This sort of balance does not result in neutralization, but instead offers additive effects that make for a relaxing stimulation—guests will be comfortable but interested.

The wines are chosen to produce a tranquility that will

take the edge off the stimulant cheese and chocolate. The brandy has a strong taste, sensory stimulation, and a high alcohol content which induces a slight feeling of well-being. The overall dinner is relatively light; larger quantities tend to induce sleep by stimulating many of the digestive processes.

In this case there is a deliberate avoidance of the spicy, communal-type serving which would stimulate animal consciousness. Similarly, substances like bananas, nutmeg, and avocado which might induce different states of consciousness are avoided.

The Romantic and Sensual Dinner for Two— A Case Study

Craig, a 34-year-old lawyer, divorced for six months following a ten-year marriage, has thrown himself into his work over the past year as his marriage has fallen apart. He has retreated from interpersonal relationships and except for an occasional date has had, up until the past two weeks, very little interest in women. Two weeks ago he passed a dark-haired young woman who was photographing children in a park. Their eyes met as he passed her; he was overpowered by something that she emanated and he stopped short. Shyly he approached her and after talking for a while they made a date. He has since gone out with her three times and cannot get her out of his mind. His days are happier and he catches himself singing when nobody is around. He is feeling again for the first time in a year, and his passion has awakened. He has invited her to his apartment for dinner and wishes to make his intimate dinner party as romantic as possible.

She is Janine, of French-American parents, and is 26 years old. She is a commercial artist who dreams of a career in photojournalism. Six months ago she parted from a friend with whom she had lived for three years, feeling that they were no longer communicating and he could not share her excitement and vision. The parting was difficult and she has lingering feelings for her former friend. She was considering responding to his request that they try to work things out when she met a man in the park as she was photographing children. She was struck by him and has been thinking of him quite a bit, but she still feels guarded even though Craig seems like a sincere and good person. She has enjoyed their first three dates, but there has been little physical contact. She feels desire, but fears at the same time. With mixed feelings she has accepted his offer of dinner at his apartment.

Craig is worried. He is falling in love and wants to woo and win this woman. It has been too long since he had a close physical relationship and he has lost much of his confidence with women. Craig is not a schemer but he wants to plan carefully for his guest.

Party Plan

The idea is to stimulate romance, delicate and loving sensuality, dissolve the rational/intellectual fears and guards that are between them, and allow comfort so they can relate as man and woman instead of as two fearful, guarded people.

Setting

His apartment has a large living room which substitutes as a dining room. It is on the twentieth floor and overlooks the city. The kitchen is small and Spartan so he decides to set his table close to the window in his living room. He will not light the entire room because that will destroy some of the intimacy. He plans to use candles and one small amber light. He stays away from white and yellow lights, knowing amber is softer, as is candlelight. The settings for the table are a delicate beige pattern. He stays away from green, a nervous color, and from red, which is too intense for now. He uses his best dishes which are a deep blue on white, and he has good silver and fine crystal wine goblets which he has recently purchased, thinking of her. There should be wine for a toast, and for this dinner the toast that comes to his mind is "To love." There are other toasts that are charming and special; he thinks of one he heard from a retired English general who had traveled widely—"To astonishing fortune."

Craig is wearing loose clothing—dark brown (a color associated with physical ease and sensuous contentment)— and he is wearing no jewelry. He has not put on his watch (something he has not done in a year), wanting this evening to have a pure and timeless quality. He wants this evening to be of them—not reminiscent of his past marriage or her past relationship.

The music in the background is instrumental, although he could also play a vocal—an emotional singer on an album about love. He puts on a tape that will reverse so he won't have to think of changing it.

The Menu

Craig knows that he wants a dinner that is easy to eat so that they won't spend most of the time struggling to cut meat or trying to get spaghetti on a fork without dropping it. Initially he had thought of some unusual cheeses to start off the evening, but he thinks the stimulation from the tyramine in the cheese might make them uncomfortable at first. However, he wants an appetizer that will not be heavy and make them drowsy or sluggish.

It is winter and he knows that when she arrives she might be a bit cold from the walk. He is very nervous and he suspects that she will be too. He decides that the first thing he should have ready is a fine bottle of Burgundy wine, which is warming and calming.

His deep-violet velour couch is in the corner with a little table for the wine glasses. He plans to have several varieties of mushrooms, which he knows she likes, and a cream cheese dip on the table. The mushrooms have long been a fertility symbol and their shape is sensual. He uses a small amount of garlic in the dip for its gentle mouth-stimulant actions. The cream cheese contains a little tryptophan which, in this small quantity, will not be sleep-inducing. The mayonnaise in the dip, made with egg, also tends to be calming because of its choline and lecithin content. These also go into the formation of acetylcholine, a glandular stimulant. A small amount of freshly ground pepper offers some additional mild stimulation.

For the main course, he chooses a seafood dish that is a mixture of scallops, oysters, and shrimp. The seafood has steroidlike substances which are sensual stimulators. The iodine's thyroid-stimulant actions will not be felt until days later, if at all. Zinc, which has been associated with male and female sexuality, is highest in seafood and particularly oysters. The seafood sauce is a white sauce with a small amount of Cheddar cheese. The cheese offers some stimulus to talk, as well as offsetting some possible effects of the wine and the tryptophan in the cream cheese and the calming effect of fats and the egg.

He has prepared an interesting salad with several different types of lettuce. The effect of the lactucin is slightly calming. He has baked his own bread and has used untreated poppy seeds; they also produce a very mild, calming contentment.

For dessert, he has prepared a chocolate fondue made from pure chocolate. He knows that chocolate has come down through history as a sexual exciter (Montezuma would not visit any of his wives without it) and that it has more than stimulant effect—it produces a slight euphoria. Pieces of fruit are there to be dipped. He chooses apples as one type because of the tradition of Eve's apple. He also has seedless grapes, which have been associated with sensual experiences. In addition, a fondue is something they both dip into—a sharing experience.

SUMMARY OF MENU:

1. French Burgundy wine
   Mushrooms
   Cream cheese–mayonnaise dip with garlic, salt, pepper
2. Main Course: seafood—scallops, oysters, shrimp in
   a white sauce made with Cheddar cheese
   Salad: varieties of lettuce
   Bread: home-baked, with poppy seeds
3. Dessert: chocolate fondue with fruit to dip—apples
   and grapes

The dinner was by soft candlelight. Janine came to Craig's apartment and was fearful and shy. Instead of an imposing lawyer's study she found a soft, playful, timeless, enchanting feeling. She was pleased by the candlelight. When she saw the fine French Burgundy she felt an inner smile and knew he had been thinking of her. The pharmacologic actions of the foods blended together to produce a calm feeling of well-being. The setting and planned menu softened the barriers between them so that they could relate on many different levels. The evening was for both love and "astonishing fortune."

The Mystical Experience and a Seance

The mystical experience is characterized by enhanced psychic awareness and spirituality. The Zen ideal, for example, is to achieve satori, which involves an intuitive looking into the nature of things as opposed to an analytical understanding. This type of "seeing" is the sort Don Juan tried to teach his pupil Carlos Castañeda. A famous Zen teacher called satori "the removal of the mind bars and the opening of the mind flower." This state of consciousness can be thought of as the superconsciousness, as contrasted with the rational/analytical consciousness and the instinctual/animal consciousness. Mystics consider it to be the illuminated consciousness, similar to highly religious states. Ancient lore describes it as being related to the third eye, which we now know as the pineal gland.

To begin, the guests should be asked to wear simple, loose-fitting clothing. If some traditional Eastern practices are followed, the guests should be asked at the door to cleanse their thoughts and ask whether they are worthy to enter. The table should be set in an orderly fashion but with the simplest of wooden implements. Chairs should be simple; floor cushions are suitable. Lighting should be subdued and red should be avoided—it is felt to incite the passions. Usually amber is the best choice, with a few touches of blue or violet.

Wordless background music of a delicate Oriental or Indian type would also help the set. Because the nondominant side of the brain (associated with intuitive phenomena) should be stimulated, the music should have low tones with complex sounds and chords, as opposed to music with a strong melody. There should be suitable books around for the guests to peruse on subjects like the I-Ching, psychic phenomena, and the occult. A deck of Tarot cards can be on a table.

Prior to eating the guests can be aided in developing their mystical consciousness by reading the Tarot cards. Or perhaps a guest can be given some object from the table and asked if he or she can re-create the place from which it came.

Some wine can be served initially—preferably a non-sparkling red wine such as a Bordeaux.

The food should be passed from person to person. Slow eating with careful chewing is helpful in delicate sensory stimulation. There should be no animal protein (meat) among the food. Aged cheeses, pickled herring, and other talk foods mentioned in chapter 9 should be avoided since nonverbal interactions are to be encouraged. The food should be vegetarian and fresh. Foods rich in serotonin or tryptophan should be chosen—nuts, dates, figs, and bananas are some choices. Fruits such as the pomegranate and mango would also be good. A variety of lettuce, and celery with alfalfa sprouts are good as salad choices. A simple vegetarian main dish employing natural rice is a good idea. Parsley can be sprinkled on it lightly and some saffron can aid the consciousness.

For beverages, an assortment of teas will enhance the desired consciousness. Some Oriental green teas, mild catnip tea, and hops tea are effective. For dessert, some simple cakes—perhaps with a message baked inside—will add to the mood. Nutmeg sprinkled on the cakes might enhance the desired state.

Certain things common at parties should be avoided. No sugar or very sweet food should be served, and it is best to avoid coffee.

A Jolly Celebration

For jolly times, people should have fun, laugh a lot, and find the absurdity in just about everything. The ideal is for guests to say, "I can't remember laughing so much."

For this there is a need to stimulate all types of consciousness, but particularly the animal/instinctual and the psychic superconsciousness. The rational/analytical should not be dominant as it tends to be too critical.

Perhaps a costume-party motif could be useful. The lighting should be of a variety of shapes and colors. Music should be designed to shift from one style to another. Decorations should include surprises—unusual and even bizarre types. Plates can be different colors and sizes. Incongruities should be about—balloons set against serious paintings is one idea.

Initially there should be free-flowing champagne, stimulant wines or beers, and platters of a wide variety of bite-sized tidbits. Overall, the food should not need excessive cutting or use of utensils since this tends to reduce social communication.

Surprise courses such as flaming dishes, or fondues with a variety of crackers and breads are good choices. Choose herbs and spices known for their stimulant effects, such as borage, saffron, nutmeg, and pepper.

It is important to stay away from things like thick steaks which require so much work to cut and result in a heavy, torpid state. More manageable meats like spareribs with diverse seasonings are suitable.

Jokes should abound and no subject matter should be taboo. The principal objective is to allow your guests to let go and play as children without self-consciousness, to be able to express emotions freely, and to revel in the beauty and absurdity of human problems and interactions that might in other settings result in serious, heavy, and earth-grounding critical discussion.

The major means of achieving this objective is through myriad and incongruous sensory stimulations, through foods and drinks that provoke talk and laughter, and by providing a free, nonthreatening environment where people can be themselves without fear.

14 Diet for the Future

Our society and the world are changing faster than at any other time in human history. These changes are happening to men and women who still have many of the basic nervous system responses of the hunter. In terms of the history of the world, our civilization is still very young. Millions of years of evolution finally produced Neanderthal man, a relatively crude hunter with a primitive capacity for what we think of as civilization. About thirty thousand years ago, Neanderthal man disappeared for no known reason and Cro-Magnon man developed. Dr. Robert Ardrey believes that the "new man" killed off the Neanderthal and cannibalized him. Perhaps this particular diet aided the evolution of man in some way. At any rate, ten thousand years ago the ice sheet which had existed for tens of thousands of years began to recede and the stage was set for the development of agriculture and a relatively stable nonhunting society.

Many of the bodily responses developed during these early stages of human evolution are unnecessary and, in fact, sometimes disease producing in our current world, yet we still retain them. For example, someone makes us angry. The adrenalin begins to flow and our bodies gear toward either attack or flight. We usually do neither and become frustrated and upset.

Diet can play a role in helping us control body responses that occur in the province of the involuntary, or autonomic, nervous system. Before describing which diets can aid this nervous system control it is important to understand more about the autonomic nervous system.

The autonomic nervous system is concerned with body events not usually under conscious control. One branch, the parasympathetic, is involved primarily with housekeeping functions—processes of digestion, glandular secretions, temperature control, urine formation, sleep, etc.

The other branch, the sympathetic, can be looked on as a protector of the body.

Walter Cannon, who was a noted physician, scientist, and philosopher, clarified much of what we know about the sympathetic nervous system. He termed it the system that gets the person ready for "fight or flight," and considered its reactions the "wisdom of the body."

The sympathetic nervous system has much to do with the adrenal gland and the flow of adrenalin. While this system induces a state of alertness, even hyperalertness and vigilance, the parasympathetic nervous system has more to do with sleep and relaxed, receptive and unprotected states. The balance between these two systems depends on many factors, mainly the person's basic constitution, age, and environmental influences.

Prolonged overactivity of the adrenal (sympathetic) system results in what Dr. Hans Selye considered the General Adaptation Syndrome—which ends with exhaustion. Prolonged underactivity results in lethargy. Foods have a good deal to do with keeping our involuntary nervous system in balance.

Often-heard expressions in our language reflect the common understanding of the balance between the sympathetic and parasympathetic nervous systems.

"Eat your heart out"—sympathetic excess
"Pain in the neck"—tightened neck muscles and pos-
     sibly increased blood pressure;
     sympathetic excess
"Feeling uptight"—sympathetic excess with constipa-
     tion
"So scared he did it in his pants"—excess bowel ac-
     tion; parasympath-
     etic excess
"Don't make me sick"—trying to avoid parasympath-
     etic excess
"Don't get your bowels in an uproar"—avoiding para-
     sympathetic
     excess

How are foods involved in the parasympathetic or sympathetic nervous systems?

The major body chemical having to do with the parasympathetic nervous system is called acetylcholine and is related to the amount of choline in our diet. A high-choline food such as egg yolks would tend to increase formation of acetylcholine.

The chemicals in the body relating to the sympathetic nervous system are adrenalinelike and arise from the amino acids phenylalanine and tyrosine. Tyrosine is also closely associated with the thyroid hormone which has resulatory functions in metabolism. Aged cheese and tyramine-wines, sugar, and other foods high in tyrosine tend to increase activity of the sympathetic nervous system.

A food such as red meat with high choline and high tyrosine tends to be involved with both.

Diet for Balance

Because of the great importance of correct balance, foods should be considered as they affect one part or the other of the autonomic nervous system. Diets rich in sympathetic stimulants will tend toward bad digestion, hyperalert states, and anxiety. Those with parasympathetic stimulants will tend toward sleepiness, increased secretions, and lethargy.

Most food charts contain information about the protein content of various foods. But just knowing the total protein does not allow us to determine the amino acid content. When thinking in terms of food power this becomes important. Decreasing the activity of the sympathetic nervous system has a calming effect. Fasting will cause such decreased activity, but on a longer-term basis fasting is obviously not an answer. What a person can do is eat foods that have protein but relatively less phenylalanine and tyrosine, or have a diet with somewhat less protein in it.

For example, milk is a protein-rich food, but in terms of phenylalanine and tyrosine, goat's milk has less than half the amount contained in cow's milk. Cheese is high in phenylalanine and tyrosine, and could be avoided. Most meats are high in these amino acids, but lamb has less than beef and pork has even less than lamb. Cereals made with buckwheat flour have lower amounts than those made from wheat or barley. Rice flour has a lower content than wheat. Fruits have relatively little and, except perhaps for bananas, all can be eaten. Of the vegetables, a person should avoid peas and beans; the lowest amounts are in the leafy vegetables.

Thus, to decrease the tyrosine and phenylalanine in a diet and, as a result, decrease the activity of the sympathetic nervous system, a person should have:

DIET 1: Suppressing the Sympathetic Nervous System

1. Lamb or pork, if meat is eaten
2. Breads made from buckwheat and rice flour
3. Fruits
4. Leafy vegetables
5. Fish in moderation

On the other hand, someone in a highly physical situation such as competitive athletics should have a diet such as:

DIET 2: Stimulating the Sympathetic Nervous System

1. Cow's milk and cheeses
2. Beef, liver, turkey
3. Whole wheat breads
4. Peas, beans, and other legumes

How can this knowledge of foods and the autonomic nervous system be further used?

Let's take the example of Dave, an ordinarily well-balanced man of 35. He has recently come to work for a nursing school as the program coordinator. Usually this is not a high-stress job, but the dean of the school in this instance is a demanding woman and Dave finds that he becomes very frustrated in his job. Every time he tries to take some independent action he is thwarted and becomes angry, but doesn't express it because he wants to keep his job and he sees changes in the future. During the time of great frustration and anger he should switch to Diet 1 (above) which will tend to decrease his body response to his frustration. If he doesn't, he will not only feel more distress, but will run the risk of acquiring a disorder associated with hyperactivity of the sympathetic nervous system, such as anxiety or hypertension.

What about the other branch of the autonomic nervous system? The parasympathetic component must also be considered in a diet of the future. Diet can particularly influence the glandular response. For example, another effect of Dave's situation of anger and frustration is an increase of cholinergic (or parasympathetic) stimulation which tends to increase his secretion of acid and stomach juices. This might give him indigestion or even an ulcer. If this occurs, the job is literally

making him sick. The parasympathetic nervous system depends to some extent on the amount of choline in his diet.
Choline is found in fatty foods and many others, including
egg yolks, meat, legumes, and wheat cereals (more than in
rice cereals). Therefore, the same diet that would suppress
the sympathetic nervous system will also suppress the parasympathetic, with one exception—fatty foods. So in addition
to following Diet 1, Dave could reduce his chances of
developing an ulcer by reducing his intake of fats.

The diet Dave should follow would avoid sympathetic
nervous system stimulants like coffee, aged cheese, red wine
and other alcoholic beverages, and reduce his overall autonomic nervous system responses. Such use of food power to
help control nervous system responses is an example of a
diet for the future.

The above case illustrates an important and basic principle of a diet for the future—the diet is for the individual
and his situation and desired state.

When considering diet to help balance the autonomic
nervous system, the basic constitution of the person has to
be considered. Just as there are short people and tall people,
people with different colored eyes and hair, there are also
people with different types of nervous systems. Everybody
knows sympathetic nervous system people ("adrenergs") who
tend to be thin, tense, and prone to anxiety attacks. A lot of
people also know somebody who is a parasympathetic nervous
system type ("cholinerg"). Such people tend to be heavier,
moody, subject to depressions or mood swings. Most people
are balanced somewhere between these extremes. Adrenerg
types should recognize themselves and seek a diet with more
choline (found in fatty foods and egg yolks) and less sympathetic nervous system stimulants. Those cholinergs should
choose a diet with reduced choline. Such people often find
that a period of fasting acts as a potent mood stabilizer.

Diet for Older People

The autonomic nervous system balance is not constant throughout a person's life, and observing changes as aging occurs provides a basis for a special diet for the elderly. First, it is important that older people ensure adequate vitamin and mineral intake. Then the diet should focus on offsetting some of the physiological changes that occur in aging. One of the most important changes is in the autonomic nervous system where there is a tendency to shift the balance more toward the sympathetic side, although the responsivity of both branches is reduced. With the shift in balance comes a decreased need for sleep and a tendency for decreased learning ability and forgetfulness. When a drug was given experimentally to elderly people that blocked the sympathetic nervous system, learning of new material improved markedly. Putting an older person on potent medication is dangerous; a better way of influencing the same thing is through food.

The diet of older people should have reduced amounts of foods that stimulate the sympathetic nervous system, including coffee, and tyramine-containing foods such as aged cheese, pickled herring, and fermented foods (see chart on page 42). Meat intake should be reduced since the amino acids tyrosine and phenylalanine go into the chemical makeup of adrenalin substances. Fish should not be excessive because the iodine is thyroid stimulating. Vegetables to stay away from include beans, peas, and seaweed. Pepper, nutmeg, monosodium glutamate, vanilla, caraway, coriander, peppermint, and thyme are seasonings to avoid.

The diet should contain (not limited to only these, but the following seem particularly important):

VEGETABLES	FRUITS	HERBS	EGGS/DAIRY PRODUCTS
lettuce	anise	rosemary	eggs (for the
celery	pineapple	dill	choline)

VEGETABLES	FRUITS	HERBS	POULTRY/FISH
carrots	mangoes	parsley	chicken
yams	pomegranates	garlic	oysters
	palm kernels	basil	shellfish
	watermelon	ginger	

FOODS TO HELP BALANCE THE NERVOUS SYSTEM

whole grain cerals
wheat germ
moderate amounts of saltwater fish
seed oils
peanuts

Using food power, we can see the objectives of a diet for the elderly:

1. Avoid excess stimulatory foods.
2. Avoid excess sleep-inducing foods.
3. Use choline foods to stimulate acetylcholine and the parasympathetic nervous system to help offset the shift in balance to the sympathetic nervous system.

Food Power Effects

When considering the effects of different foods, both the direct and indirect effects must be considered. The direct effect results from a druglike action of a substance like the caffeine in coffee.

An indirect effect results when a food is taken that stimulates a body response. For example, sugar will stimulate insulin, and the effects of sugar in most people include an initial stimulation followed by a letdown hours later as the insulin response lowers the blood sugar. Another indirect effect comes when a substance necessary to make a hormone or body compound is taken. For example, iodine has little effect by itself, but as a stimulant to the formation of thyroid hormone it can effect a later change. Choline and the amino acids phenylalanine and tyrosine are similar in that they are the building blocks of other body substances.

Mixed effects (direct and indirect) are most common. For example, a person eats a plate of oysters. The hormonelike effects can be seen within hours, and the effects of the amino acids, proteins, and iodine within days.

Diet for Consciousness

A diet for the future must take man's varieties of consciousness into consideration. We are not always the same way—none of us are—and different diets and meals can take these into account. Let's briefly explore each state.

The Animal Consciousness

This is instinctual and seeks gratification on an immediate basis. Sexual feelings are included here in their most primitive state. A baby has primarily an animal consciousness. The person with the animal consciousness exists for the moment; past and future are not important. Certain foods may help to stimulate this state (e.g., a barbecued whole leg of lamb, a communal pot of spaghetti with a spicy hot red sauce). Settings to induce this consciousness are designed to lower boundaries between people.

The Rational/Intellectual Consciousness

This is the consciousness of the contemporary business world or scientific world—analytical, critical, worldly, highly factual, formal. There is usually talk, but it concerns external events such as elections, politics, the economy, etc. The type of setting and foods that stimulate this consciousness are those with clear definition—discrete, formal food courses, talk foods, and unromantic atmosphere.

The Superconsciousness

This is more intuitive. Talk tends to relate to perceptions, intuitions, and feelings. Religious states are within this category as are aspects of creative states. Feelings of love—not lust—are part of the superconsciousness. The superconscious individual can experience a cosmic consciousness, which is a feeling of unity with others and the universe. Foods involved in religious and creative states and, to some extent, high-powered foods facilitate this consciousness.

The Mystical Realms

These are the realms of the superconsciousness taken to their ecstatic extreme. Such states seem to relate to a third type of nervous system located within the brain. When dealing with this we come full-front with the mind-brain relationship. Wilder Penfield, a neurosurgeon and one of the leading brain researchers of our time, concluded soon before his death that there is something which we term the mind not found within the brain. The brain is the organ that does the work but the essential person, the "I," is not the brain. Thus there is something not of the body which is a person's essence. Religious people call this the soul.

The experience in the highest state of consciousness—the transcendent experience, the conversion experience, or the visionary experience—can be imitated through the high-powered food-drugs such as psilocybin mushrooms and peyote cactus. The mediation of such experiences seems to involve a substance in the brain called serotonin. Perhaps it also relates to the pineal gland, or "inner eye."

Many of these states have been reported after fasting and isolation along with intensive meditation and quieting of the brain activity. Foods other than the high-powered food-drugs seem to relate to this state negatively. Since all foods are chemicals, the entry of any external foodstuff would tend to produce some changes to offset the mental quiescence which seems to be a prerequisite for reaching this particular state of consciousness.

It is ironic that food power can be used to assist all the other activities of our being, from sleep to creativity to conversation to comfort. But the most ineffable experience, the most unique and esoteric state of mind, is best reached through the absence of food.

Bibliography

In this bibliography only the most useful books are listed. The bibliography of articles numbers over three thousand and is available to any reader upon request.

American Can Company, Research Division: *The Canned Food Reference Manual*, American Can Company, New York, 1949.

Apt, C., ed.: *Flavor: Its Chemical, Behavioral and Commercial Aspects*, Westview Press, Boulder, Col., 1977.

Ardrey, R.: *African Genesis*, Atheneum, New York, 1961.

————: *The Hunting Hypothesis*, Atheneum, New York, 1976.

Atkins, Robert C.: *Protein for Vegetarians*, Pyramid Publications, New York, 1976.

Barbeau, A., and R. Huxtable, eds.: *Taurine and Neurological Disorders*, Raven Press, New York, 1978.

Berg, Alan: *The Nutrition Factor*, The Brookings Institution, Washington, D.C., 1973.

Berglund, B., and Clare Bolsby: *Edible Wild Plants*, Charles Scribner's Sons, New York, 1977.

Bolitho, Hector: *The Glorious Oyster*, Sidgwick and Jackson, London, 1960.

Born, Wina: *The Concise Atlas of Wine*, Charles Scribner's Sons, New York, 1972.

Brecher, Edward M.: *Licit and Illicit Drugs*, Little, Brown and Company, Boston, 1972.

Breeling, J. L. and M. Nagy: *Symposium on Newer Food Processing Technology*, American Medical Association Publication, 1973.

Campbell, Hannah: *Why Did They Name It . . . ?*, Bell Publishing Company, New York, 1964.

Campbell, J., ed.: *The Portable Jung*, The Viking Press, New York, 1971.

Castañeda, Carlos: *The Teachings of Don Juan: A Yaqui Way of Knowledge*, Simon & Schuster, New York, 1973.

Cheraskin, E., W. M. Ringsdorf, Jr., and Arline Brecher: *Psychodietetics*, Bantam Books, New York, 1974.

Ciba Foundation Symposium 22 (New Series): *Aromatic Amino Acids in the Brain*, Associated Scientific Publishers, Amsterdam, 1974.

Conway, David: *The Magic of Herbs*, E. P. Dutton and Company, New York, 1976.

Coon, C. S.: *The Hunting Peoples*, Little, Brown and Company, Boston, 1971.

Crow, W. B.: *The Occult Properties of Herbs*, Samuel Weiser, New York, 1969.

Davies, David: *The Centenarians of the Andes*, Anchor Press/Doubleday, Garden City, N.Y., 1975.

Davis, Adelle: *Let's Eat Right to Keep Fit*, Harcourt Brace Jovanovich, New York, 1970.

Davison, A. N., ed.: *Biochemical Correlates of Brain Structure and Function*, Academic Press, New York, 1977.

Draper, Harold: *Advances in Nutritional Research*, Plenum Press, New York, 1977.

Eccles, J.: *The Physiology of Nerve Cells*, Johns Hopkins University Press, Baltimore, 1957.

Eccles, John: *The Understanding of the Brain*, McGraw-Hill Book Company, New York, 1973.

Evans, T., and D. Greene: *The Meat Book*, Charles Scribner's Sons, New York, 1973.

Evers, N., and D. Caldwell: *The Chemistry of Drugs*, Interscience Publishers, Inc., New York, 1959.

Freedland, R. A., and S. Briggs: *A Biochemical Approach to Nutrition*, John Wiley and Sons, New York, 1977.

Freud, S.: *Beyond the Pleasure Principle*, W. W. Norton and Company, New York, 1961.

Fryer, L., and A. Dickinson: *A Dictionary of Food Supplements*, Mason-Charter, New York, 1975.

Galli, C., G. Jacini, and A. Pecile, eds.: *Dietary Lipids and Postnatal Development*, Raven Press, New York, 1973.

Gellhorn, E., *Autonomic Regulations*, Interscience, New York, 1943.
———, and G. Loofbourrow: *Emotions and Emotional Disorders*, Harper & Row, New York, 1963.

Goodhart, R. S., and M. E. Shills: *Modern Nutrition in Health and Disease Dietotherapy*, Lea and Febiger, Philadelphia, 1973.

Goodman, L. S., and A. Gilman: *The Pharmacologic Basis of Therapeutics*, The Macmillan Company, New York, 1975.

Hall, R. H.: *Food for Nought*, Vintage Books, New York, 1976.

Harris, B. C.: *Kitchen Medicines*, Pocket Books, New York, 1970.

Harris, M.: *Cannibals and Kings,* Random House, New York, 1977.

Harris, R. S., and H. Von Loldcke, eds.: *Nutritional Evaluation of Food Processing,* Avi Publishing, Westport, Conn., 1971.

Hathcock, J. N., and J. Coon: *Nutrition and Drug Interrelations,* Academic Press, New York, 1978.

Hill, H.: *Ninety-Nine Miracle Food Products of Nature,* Castle Books, Secaucus, New Jersey, 1973.

Himwich, H. E., ed.: *Brain Metabolism and Cerebral Disorders,* Spectrum Publications, New York, 1976.

Hoagland, H.: *Hormones, Brain Function and Behavior,* Academic Press, New York, 1957.

Hudson, P.: *Mastering Herbalism,* Stein and Day, New York, 1974.

Humphey, S. W.: *Spices, Seasonings and Herbs,* The Macmillan Company, New York, 1965.

Hur, Robin: *Food Reform: Our Desperate Need,* Heidelberg Publishing, Austin, Tex., 1973.

Huxley, Aldous: *Doors of Perception*, Harper & Row, New York, 1954.

Huxley, Anthony: *Plant and Planet,* The Viking Press, New York, 1975.

Kazin, A.: *Writers at Work,* The Viking Press, New York, 1967.

Koestler, A.: *The Act of Creation,* Dell, New York, 1964.

Kordel, L.: *Eat and Grow Younger,* Manor Books, New York, 1976.

————: *Natural Folk Remedies,* Manor Books, New York, 1976.

Kutsky, R.: *Handbook of Vitamins and Hormones,* Van Nostrand Reinhold Company, New York, 1973.

Lehane, B.: *The Power of Plants,* McGraw-Hill, Maidenhead, England, 1977.

Lilliston, L.: *Mega-Vitamins: A New Key to Health,* Fawcett Publications, Greenwich, Conn., 1975.

Lott, A.: *Fasting: The Ultimate Diet,* Bantam Books, New York, 1975.

Lucas, Jack: *Our Polluted Food,* Charles Knight and Company, London, 1975.

Lucra, S.: *Medicinal Uses of Wine,* Wine Advisory Board of California, 1972.

Lüscher, M.: *The Lüscher Color Test,* Random House, New York, 1969; Pocket Books, New York, 1971.

Milton, John: "Paradise Lost," in M. H. Abrams, gen. ed., *The*

Norton Anthology of English Literature, W. W. Norton and Company, New York, 1962.

Muenscher, W. C.: *Poisonous Plants of the United States,* The Macmillan Company, New York, 1964.

Myers, F. H., E. Jawetz, and A. Goldfien: *Review of Medical Pharmacology,* Lange Medical Publishers, Los Altos, Calif., 1974.

Myers, R. D.: *Handbook of Drug and Chemical Stimulation of the Brain,* Van Nostrand Reinhold Company, New York, 1974.

Norman, Barbara: *Tales of the Table,* Prentice-Hall, Englewood Cliffs, N.J., 1972.

Null, G.: *Protein for Vegetarians,* Pyramid Books, New York, 1976.

———, and S. Null: *The Complete Book of Nutrition,* Dell, New York, 1972.

Okakura, Kakuzo: *The Book of Tea,* Dover Publications, New York, 1964.

Osler, W.: *The Principles and Practice of Medicine,* D. Appleton, New York, 1919.

Ouspensky, P. D.: *The Fourth Way,* Vintage Books, New York, 1971.

Packard, V.: *Processed Foods and the Consumer,* University of Minnesota Press, Minneapolis, 1976.

Parsons, J. A., ed.: *Peptide Hormones,* University Park Press, Baltimore, 1976.

Pearce, J. C.: *The Crack in the Cosmic Egg,* Pocket Books, New York, 1971.

Perry, Francis, ed.: *Complete Guide to Plants and Flowers,* Simon & Schuster, New York, 1974.

Potter, S. O.; Scott, R. J. E., *Therapeutics, Materia Medica and Pharmacy,* P. Blackiston's Son and Co., Philadelphia, 1926.

Prasad, J., et al.: *Zinc and Man,* Charles C Thomas, Springfield, Ill., 1966.

Prescott, J. W., M. S. Read, and D. B. Coursin: *Brain Function and Malnutrition,* John Wiley and Sons, New York, 1975.

Quimme, P.: *Coffee and Tea,* Signet Books, New York, 1976.

Rechcigl, Miloslav: *Man, Food and Nutrition,* CRC Press, Cleveland, Oh., 1973.

Rolleston, H. D.: *The Endocrine Organs in Health and Disease,* Oxford Press, London, 1936.

Schlesinger, A. M.: *Paths to the Present,* The Macmillan Company, New York, 1949.

Schultes, R.: *Hallucinogenic Plants*, Golden Press, New York, 1976.

Selye, Hans: *Stress in Health and Disease*, Butterworth, Boston, 1976.

Serban, G., ed.: *Nutrition and Mental Functions*, Plenum Press, New York, 1975.

Shakespeare, W.: *The Complete Works*, Avenel Books, New York, 1975.

———, *Othello*, J. R. Brown, ed., Harcourt Brace Jovanovich, New York, 1973.

Shalleck, J.: *Tea*, The Viking Press, New York, 1971.

Sherrington, C. S.: *The Integrative Action of the Nervous System*, Yale University Press, New Haven, Conn., 1906.

Sigerist, H. E.: *A History of Medicine*, Vol. I, Oxford Press, London, 1951.

Simmons, A. G.: *Herb Gardens of Delight*, Hawthorne Books, New York, 1974.

Stafford, P.: Psychedelics Encyclopedia and/or Press, Berkeley, Calif., 1977.

Stecher, P. G., et al.: *The Merck Index*, Eighth Ed., Merck and Co., Inc., Rahway, N.J., 1968.

Still, H.: *Of Time, Tides and Inner Clocks*, Pyramid Books, New York, 1975.

Stillé, A.: *Therapeutics and Materia Medica*, Henry C. Lea, Philadelphia, 1874.

Tannahil, Reay: *Food in History*, Stein and Day, New York, 1973.

Teilhard de Chardin, Pierre: *Building the Earth*, Avon, New York, 1965.

Toffler, A.: *Future Shock*, Random House, New York, 1970.

Waite, A. E.: *The Holy Kabbalah*, University Books, Secaucus, N.J., 1960.

Walcher, D. N., N. Kretchmer, and H. L. Barnett: *Food, Man and Society*, Plenum Press, New York, 1976.

Wason, B.: *Encyclopedia of Cheese and Cheese Cookery*, Galahad Books, New York, 1966.

Weil, Andrew: *The Natural Mind*, Houghton Mifflin, Boston, 1972.

Wheelwright, E. G.: *Medicinal Plants and Their History*, Dover Publications, New York, 1974.

White, J., ed.: *The Highest State of Consciousness*, Anchor Books, New York, 1972.

Wilson, C. O., and O. Grisvold: *Textbook of Organic Medical and Pharmaceutical Chemistry,* J. B. Lippincott, Philadelphia, 1956.

Wurtman, R. J., and J. J. Wurtman, eds.: *Nutrition and the Brain,* Vols. I and II, Raven Press, New York, 1977.

Yu Lu, *The Classic of Tea,* Little, Brown and Company, Boston, 1974.